TYPHOID MA

TYPHOID MARY

An Urban Historical

by

Anthony Bourdain

BLOOMSBURY

Published by Bloomsbury, New York and London
Distributed to the trade by St. Martin's Press

Library of Congress Cataloging-in-Publication Data

Bourdain, Anthony.
Typhoid Mary: an urban historical / by Anthony Bourdain.
p. cm.
Includes bibliographical references.
ISBN 1-58234-133-8
1. Typhoid Mary, d. 1938. 2. Typhoid fever--New York
(State)--New York--History. 3. Quarantine--New York
(State)--New York--History. I. Title.

RA644.T8 B68 2001
614.5′112′097471092--dc21
[B] 2001018444

First U.S. Edition

10 9 8 7 6 5 4 3 2

Typeset by Hewer Text Ltd, Edinburgh, Scotland
Printed and bound in the United States of America
by R.R. Donnelley & Sons

to Nancy

'God sends us meat –
but the devil sends us cooks.'

– Julius Chambers from *The Book of New York*
quoting an unnamed 'grouchy Englishman'

Author's Prologue

Sick

HISTORICALLY, TO BE A COOK, to prepare food for others, was always to identify oneself with the degraded and the debauched. As far back as ancient Rome, and as recently as pre-Civil War America, cooks were slaves. Untrustworthy, unpleasant, and more often than not, unhealthy, cooks in early twentieth-century Europe and America worked in hot, unventilated spaces for long hours. They were underpaid, underfed, and underappreciated – their cruel masters despotic, megalomaniacal tyrants, parsimonious desk-jockeys, and brutish warders. Cooks tended – as they still do – to drink. And they died, usually at a young age, with their livers bloated by booze, their feet flattened, hands gnarled, faces ravaged, their lungs coated with the sediment of years of inhaling smoke, airborne grease, and bad air. Their brains were fried by the heat and the pressure and the difficulty of suppressing mammoth surges of rage and frustration, their nervous systems frazzled by mood swings which peaked and crashed with each incoming rush of business. They sweated and toiled in obscurity, cursed their customers, one another, their underlings, and their evil overlords. They cursed the world outside their kitchen doors for making them work like animals, for making them bend always to another's will. For existing.

And yet they were almost always proud. Cooks knew then, as they know now, that the people 'out there,' – the ones who lived outside those swinging kitchen doors, the ones who owned homes, who went out to dinner or to the theater on weekend nights, the ones who had holidays off and who saw their loved ones for more than a few fleeting hours a week, were different. Civilians, as all cooks know, take their pleasures in different ways and, just as significantly, at different times. The rules they live by are different too. And just as cooks are not understood, they don't, can't, and never have understood 'them'. The world of the nine-to-five worker, the property owner, the regular restaurant goer, the boss, is completely and maddeningly incomprehensible to those who've spent most of their lives bent over a hot range. As author Michael Ruhlman points out, cooks don't understand how others can live the way they live out there, in all that sloppy, unregimented luxury. It's messy. It's wasteful. It's scary and disorganized. *Out there*, things just don't seem to *work* the way they should.

For a cook, the well-ordered safety and certainty of the kitchen, however hot, cramped, and occasionally crazed, is a place of absolutes. The chef is the Absolute Leader. Food is always served on time. Cold food is served cold. Hot food is served hot. No one is late. No one calls in sick.

Let me repeat that: *No one* calls in sick.

The world outside the kitchen doors, to the mind of the cook, is imperfect – a constant source of disappointment, a place of thousands of tiny betrayals which threatens at all times to intrude into their own territory. Cooks are territorial creatures. No Serbian militia or feral dog defends its terrain more fiercely, and seemingly unreasonably, than a cook protects his station. *Mis-en-place*, the general sense of things being the way they should be – of being ready for anything – extends only to the exit. Outside, it's a strange and terrible place where things happen and don't happen in unpredictable and unforeseeable ways.

Mary Mallon, the woman who came (to her everlasting displeasure) to be known as Typhoid Mary, was a cook. Much has been written about Ms. Mallon over the years. There have been sensational newspaper accounts, plays, works of fiction, the predictable feminist reevaluations depicting her as the sad victim of an unfeeling, racist, sexist society bent on bringing a good woman down – her persecution and incarceration the result of some gender-insensitive Neanderthals looking for a quick fix to an embarrassing public health problem. And there is an element of truth in almost all these characterizations. She *was* a woman. She *was* Irish. She *was* poor. None of these, listed on a resume in 1906, was going to put you on the fast track to the White House or a corporate boardroom or even a box seat at the opera.

Because, first and foremost, Mary Mallon was a cook.

And her story, first and foremost, is the story of a cook. While that may not explain everything about some of the troubling aspects of her life, it explains a hell of a lot. Her tale has not yet, to my knowledge, been told from that point of view.

Little historical record of Mary's life can be depended on – and there are few recorded words or utterances from her own mouth. The accounts of the time, from others involved, directly or indirectly, with her case, are all too often self-serving, incomplete, sensationalistic, or plain wrong. Few, if any, take into account the worldview of the career cook.

There is one excellent, scrupulously researched, comprehensive and insightful telling of Mary's story: Judith Walzer Leavitt's *Typhoid Mary: Captive to the Public's Health*, an absolutely indispensable volume which should (and did, in my case) serve as a road map to anyone interested in her life and times. But Leavitt's work focuses largely on the troubling public health and civil liberties issues raised by Mary's incarceration by health authorities, drawing a meaningful comparison to today's AIDS crisis, and the moral quagmire officials encounter when confronted with otherwise blameless people who can, through casual contact with others, cause illness or death.

That's not where I'm going here. I'm a chef, and what interests me is the story of a proud cook – a reasonably capable one by all accounts – who at the outset, at least, found herself utterly screwed by forces she neither understood nor had the ability to control. I'm interested in a tormented loner, a woman in a male world, in hostile territory, frequently on the run. And I'm interested in denial – the ways that Mary, and many of us, find to avoid the obvious, the lies we tell ourselves to get through the day, the things we do and say so that we can go on, drag our aching carcasses out of bed each day, climb into our clothes and once again set out for work, often in kitchens where the smell, the surroundings, the ruling regime oppress us.

Going in, I knew only that she was a cook with a problem. Few, it seemed, knew her real name. 'Typhoid Mary', the moniker she's come to be remembered by, is now an all-purpose pejorative, an epithet implying evil intent, willful contagion; shorthand for a woman so foul, so unpleasant, so infectious as to destroy all she touches. If you were to ask a passerby who Typhoid Mary was, you might hear that she was a plague carrier, someone responsible for infecting and killing thousands.

In fact, as I soon discovered, Mary's total body count – for all her career – as tabulated by her most fervent and least forgiving pursuer – came to thirty-three persons infected, with confirmed deaths of only three. Although, in all likelihood, there probably were a few more uncounted, undiscovered cases associated with Mary. God bless her, she often worked off the books.

So knowing nothing when I began this project, I soon found myself rooting around dusty collections, library stacks and archives. Research was fun, I have to say. I've been penned up in various versions of a 25-foot by 10-foot professional kitchen (like Mary) for most of my adult life, so it was a very new experience for me to acquire knowledge in silence, seated. It helped that I was writing about a fellow cook.

The history of my profession has always fascinated me. Years ago, at culinary school, my fellow students and I loved the stories of Vatel, for instance, impaling himself on his sword over a late fish delivery. While we admired the seriousness with which he took his enterprise, we also thought, 'What a punk! Who hadda cover for him the next day at work?!' Carême's edible monuments and minarets, his kooky ambition to marry architecture, fine art, and the preparation of food inspired generations of cooks to all sorts of terrible and ludicrous excesses, nearly drove some insane trying to emulate his maniacal construction projects. We have – all of us professionals – worshipped at the altar of Escoffier, memorized his recipes, been drilled in his methods, heard and cherished stories of the Great Man, burned his image and the names of his dishes into our brains as deeply as any disciples of Chairman Mao or L. Ron Hubbard. We know the names of the greats like divinity students know the names of the apostles: Point, Troisgros, Bocuse, Guerard, Robuchon, and so on . . . We know their progeny, the ones who came after – who begot whom – and in which kitchens – and we are comforted by knowing the names. It puts our own lives, our own toil, in perspective – it reminds us that we are a part of something, cogs, however tiny, in a great machine whose wheels have been turning for centuries. One of the best parts of being a chef or a cook is exactly that sense of belonging to something, of being made members of a large and secret society. It feels good knowing you are part of a long and glorious tradition of suffering, insanity, and excess. We may not have a secret handshake (though even brushing contact with the callused hand of another cook communicates, in an instant, scads of information) but we have a language, customs, tribal rituals all our own. There is a common structure, a shared understanding of the world, a hierarchy, terminology, and initiation with which we are all – whether flipping burgers in a Bora Bora beach bar or spooning caviar at the top of the World Trade Center – intimately familiar, and we take comfort in that too.

It has been until all too recently, however, a predominantly male club, this thing of ours. In exactly the reverse of the ignorant dictum that 'Women Should Stay In The Kitchen – Preferably While Barefoot and Pregnant', in the hotel/restaurant kitchen it was always, 'They're not strong enough to lift heavy stockpots!' (Hilariously wrong in that NO cook I've ever seen hoisted full stockpots without assistance – okay, one guy. We called him Hernia Boy.) Women, it was said, 'Can't take the pressure!' they're 'Too emotional!' You want to see emotional? Watch a table of ten's order come back for a refire in a busy all-male kitchen in the middle of the rush. You've never seen such weeping and rending of garments and tantrum throwing since you smacked your little brother and took away his favorite stuffed toy.

Point is, in the annals of professional cooking, there are precious few names of women. Catherine de Medici comes to mind, but she didn't cook. She was, however, smart enough to bring along some Italian cooks when she moved to France. Had she not, the French might still be thickening their sauces with bread raspings – and tearing at their food with daggers and bare hands.

Not that women weren't cooking professionally. There were, all along, at any given moment, probably more women cooking than men. It's just that they were doing it in private homes, tiny bistros, Parisian pork stores, institutions. They stayed closer to the traditional role of professional cook of Roman times – which is to say they were slaves. Or darn close. They cooked, most times, alone. The domestic cooks of the nineteenth century and early twentieth didn't often work as part of a crew (a tendency tragically mirrored today with the predominance of the female pâtissier in the otherwise all-male kitchen). They didn't get to enjoy the yo-ho-ho camaraderie, the grab-ass hijinks of the restaurant kitchen. They did not enjoy the aid and company of sauciers, grillardins, entremetiers, poissoniers, garde-mangers, and plongeurs to assist them in their work. There were rarely chefs or souschefs to stand between them and their masters, no one to protect them from the caprices and unreasonable desires of their clients.

If Mary was part of anything, she was part of a very different movement, one forged in hunger, dislocation and social upheaval, a sea-change which pushed millions of women out of their homeland and away from their traditional roles, across the sea and into the lonely business of domestic servitude.

I have known, at various low points in my long and checkered career, what it feels like when one's pride in what one does – one's love of cooking, one's faith in one's ability – begins to fade, and I know the kind of sloppiness that can follow. Fortunately, in my case, those days are long gone. I got a second chance. Mary never did.

Bouncing from job to job, with lousy pay, no health insurance, no sick days, no vacation, miss one day at work and it's back on the treadmill . . . find another dirty, badly equipped kitchen . . . and no hope in the world. You endure simply so that you can afford to go on enduring. The small, simple joys of a perfectly made bowl of soup, a rustic stew, a lovely piece of fish cooked just right, disappear, replaced over time by a simmering forced-down resentment, bubbling up and choked down again and again like burning reflux. The small annoyances grow large: the way the boss smacks his wet lips when he tastes the soup, the acrid cloud from the steam table, the smell of old grease, the lingering odor of lamb fat – these become the nexus of all the evils and injustices of the world.

That you may have cooked good food in the past, worked in the homes of the rich, in great houses or great kitchens, seen the pyramids or danced naked on the moon, matters not at all. Nobody cares.

Where once you would have turned your head to cough, you turn no longer. Wash your hands after going to the bathroom? Maybe. If you have time, you're beyond caring. The people eating your food are abstractions now. Cough or no cough, you know they'll be back tomorrow, maybe for the Early Bird, the All-You-Can-Eat special. Unwashed hands, an errant cigarette ash, a roasted chicken dropped on a dirty kitchen floor and retrieved on the bounce . . . we've been there, you and me and Mary.

The central question when examining the career of Mary Mallon, cook, is always, 'Why did she go on cooking when she had every reason to believe she was spreading a possibly fatal disease?' Many of you who've worked in greasy spoons, coffee shops, cafeterias, failing, not-very-good restaurants, institutional food services, know the answer already. I won't blame you if you don't care to admit it. But you know what the 'three-second rule' is. Don't you?

Cooks work sick. They always have. Most jobs, you don't work, you don't get paid. You wake up with a sniffle and a runny nose, a sore throat? You soldier on. You put in your hours. You wrap a towel around your neck and you do your best to get through. It's a point of pride, working through pain and illness. And in the paranoid realpolitik world of the kitchen it makes a great deal of sense. If you don't show up to work, someone else fills in for you – either an already overburdened fellow cook, who takes on additional tasks – or worse, an outsider, an interloper, a stranger who might well be considered to do a better job than you – or be less likely to call in sick in the future. When you are working in a kitchen that serves something less than haute cuisine, the likelihood increases that a strong back and the ability to endure are of the utmost importance, a chef or owner frequently passing over the superior technician for the more reliable one.

Mary, it should be pointed out, felt fine. She was strong. She was tough. She could take it – and she was proud of her endurance. She worked, and she went on – and when after a time they told her to stop, she ignored them and went on working. One finds oneself being defined by one's job. The job expiates us from sin; it excuses us our excesses and our lapses. That we are tired, or ill, or in extremis and yet persevere is all we have, sometimes, to sustain our image of ourselves.

Like Mary, I've worked for private clients. Briefly. Had I stayed on, had my boss asked me one more time for 'an egg-white omelette – and no butter or oil in the pan,' I would surely have grabbed hold of his skull, squeezed until his eyeballs popped out of his head like pachinko balls. Had I worked in the homes of the rich and silly circa 1906? I would have murdered them in their beds with the nearest available blunt object. I was never tough enough to put up with what Mary put up with. I'm 'too emotional'; I couldn't have 'taken the pressure'; I doubt very much I could have picked up heavy stockpots alone.

Mary learned her trade over time, the same way most of us learn. By watching, waiting, working our way slowly up from the bottom. By repeating the same tasks over and over again. It's a terrible thing – the worst thing, when a good cook, a proud cook goes bad. When pride and proficiency turn to bitterness and sloth. When outside forces corrupt the desire to do a job well and take pleasure in the doing. It's an awful thing to watch. It's awful when it happens to you.

It's what happened to the cook, Mary Mallon.

Try not to hold it against her.

Chapter One

There's Something About Mary

IT WAS AUGUST 27, 1906, when at the rented summer home of Charles Henry Warren and family in Oyster Bay, Long Island, the Warrens' young daughter became ill with what was diagnosed as typhoid fever. The same week, five more persons began showing symptoms: Mrs. Warren, a second daughter, two maids, and the gardener. The relatively affluent town of Oyster Bay had never had an outbreak of typhoid before. A popular vacation spot for wealthy urban New Yorkers, it was best known for hosting President Theodore Roosevelt during the summer. The house the Warrens had taken for the season stood on high ground, overlooking the bay, and the circumstances of its occupants were impeccable – a wealthy banker, his family and their servants, living in fairly luxurious style.

The Warren family were not the type of people thought likely to contract typhoid – an illness widely associated with poverty and filth. Charles Warren was the president of the Lincoln Bank. They were the sort of folks who could afford to rent a nice big summer home on affluent Long Island (as well as hire a cook, servants, and gardener to keep things tidy). Rich people just didn't get typhoid –

especially in Oyster Bay – and predictably, there was concern in the area that the town would become a less desirable resort should it be seen as teeming with the disease.

George Thompson, the owner of the house, was particularly worried, concerned that no well-to-do New Yorkers would be of a mind to rent his home the following season if it was associated with disease. The house was very large, and expensive to run. Thompson himself, though the owner of four other homes, could not afford to live there. If the house lay vacant, it would mean disaster. Desperate, he called in experts to track down the source of the contagion, hoping it came from outside the property and eager for someone to prove it.

Drinking water was analyzed. The single indoor toilet, the cesspool, manure pit, and outhouse were all examined and ultimately rejected as the possible source of infection.

Dairy products were inspected.

An old woman who lived on the beach was considered a likely suspect. She had offered the family clams for sale, and these were scrutinized minutely, but no one else in the town who had eaten shellfish from the same source had fallen ill.

Thompson, unsatisfied with the inconclusive results from local health authorities on the scene and from his hired experts, reached out to friends in New York City, looking for someone, anyone, to help him with his embarrassing problem.

Salvation didn't exactly ride in on a white horse. Nor was Dr. George Soper hero material exactly. Dr. Soper was not even in fact a medical doctor. He was a sanitary engineer – as one newspaper described him: 'a doctor to sick cities.'

Called into the fray, he took the train out to Oyster Bay from the city and set immediately to work. After reviewing the findings of the first medical men on the scene, as well as those of earlier experts who had scrutinized the drinking water, trash and sewage, he began questioning members of the household, inquiring about visitors, ultimately receiving a comprehensive list going back an impressive ten years. To the best of his ability, Soper examined the medical histories of each of these individuals, eventually ruling all of them out as possible sources.

This was frustrating. Things usually went pretty quickly in cases like this. Feces in the water supply, contaminated milk, a sickly visitor, and case closed. Not so at the Thompson house. Soper began to 'walk the cat backward' in search of an answer.

Typhoid's incubation period was known to be ten to fourteen days long, so he focused on a time on or before August 20. Soper was intrigued by the news that on the fourth of the month, the Warrens had seen fit to change cooks. More significantly, the new cook, a Mary Mallon, was now missing, having left without notice or explanation some three weeks after the sickness began.

A missing cook! It was the kind of lead that criminal

investigators find almost *too* easy, *too* good to be true; evidence of a kind that prosecutors like to present to jurors as indicating 'guilty knowledge', the kind of red flag that Miss Marple or Hercule Poirot would disregard automatically as being just too obvious. Look at it: A murder or some other felony is committed in a household or place of business, and someone who *used to be* there is suddenly *no longer* there. It doesn't take an investigative mastermind to deduce who to go looking for first. It was circumstantial evidence of the most provocative kind, and Soper was well acquainted with the old saw about circumstantial evidence: 'It's like finding a goldfish in your milk. It doesn't prove anything – but it's mighty suspicious'.

He went over the facts of the case as they had presented themselves to him. Here he had an unexplained outbreak of typhoid in an area where no typhoid of any kind had been previously. The home was immaculate, clean from top to bottom. All other possible sources of infection had been examined and ruled out. The only new element introduced into the household had been a cook. The cook handled food, which all the afflicted members of the household had eaten. The disease broke out, and the cook was now gone. Had she left under different circumstances, say, the disappearance of a diamond necklace, the cops – or any investigator – would have been looking very hard in her direction.

Soper got a description of the suspect: a woman of

about forty, tall, with a buxom build, blond hair, blue eyes, and a firm mouth and jaw. It was remarked that she was 'a pretty good cook', though she was observed by some interviewees in retrospect as being 'not particularly clean' in her work habits and 'difficult to talk to'.

Writing later, Soper describes what he did next:

First, I went to the employment agency where I was given the missing cook's former places of employment and the different people who had furnished her with references. Working from agency to agency I came in possession of little fragments of her history for ten years. What do you suppose I found out? That in every household in which she had worked in the last ten years there had been an outbreak of typhoid fever. Mind you, there wasn't a single exception.

The question that confronted me now was: Where is she?

Following her trail backward to cases in 1904, I found she had worked at the home of Henry Gilsey at Sands Point, Long Island, where four of seven servants suddenly got the disease. Going back still further, I found that five weeks after Mary had gone to cook at the summer home of J. Coleman Drayton at Dark Harbor, Maine, in 1902, seven out of nine persons in the house contracted typhoid, and so did a trained nurse and a woman who came to the house to work by the day. There had been an outbreak of the disease in New York in

1901, and I had reason to believe that Mary was behind this. In 1904, Tuxedo Park, the fashionable summer resort, was stricken . . . and (I) discovered she had cooked there in that time.

Soper now uncovered 'other episodes', as he called them. Provocatively, there was a two-year period for which there were no records available at all for Ms. Mallon's employment – the period between the Gilsey family incident and Mary's arrival in Oyster Bay.

The two-year blank was tantalizing to Soper. Where had Mary been? Who had she been cooking for? She must have been cooking somewhere . . . The sanitary engineer's mind teemed with disturbing images. He no doubt pictured the cook stirring soup in some unknown and very busy cellar kitchen, barehanded, unknowing, infecting untold multitudes of solid citizens with potentially deadly bacilli.

Dr. Soper's breathless, self-serving, yet ultimately unreliable accounts to newspapers give a sense of how excited he was, how exhilarated by the thrill of the chase and the tantalizing prospect of being onto something really important. At first he had anticipated a case that might last only a few weeks – a little sea air, a few bowls of steamers, some resolution, and back to the city – but now he found himself further drawn into a quest which had already occupied him for a full four months. The Warrens were long gone – back home with the other summer renters. The weather had turned colder, the house now stood empty.

But George Soper was still on the case, sensing that with Mary Mallon's help, he was about to make medical history.

First of all, he realized the typhoid outbreaks associated with Mary Mallon were unusual in that they seemed to afflict the clean, well-kept houses of the affluent. While the 'filth theory' of contagion – which stated that filth, in and of itself, was the cause of disease – had been recently supplanted by the specific identification of disease-causing microbes, there was still a general sense that epidemics were closely associated with dirty living conditions and with marginal, impoverished people who lived in close, unsanitary circumstances. Many *still* held this notion, including some in the scientific community, where papers continued to be published in 1906 stating that typhoid rose up out of 'sewer gasses: and the 'miasma'. Society, for good reason, had been congratulating itself on such sensible collective widespread improvements as clean, feces-free drinking water, carefully monitored dairy products, more effective waste disposal, and new kitchen design and equipment which allowed more sanitary food handling. Congress had passed, in 1906, the Pure Food and Drug Act, and major food processors like Heinz and Kellogg's made 'purity' of food products a selling point. Sick people and people who were thought likely to be infected – such as immigrants –

were routinely detained and quarantined to avoid the possible spread of contagion. This particular situation, the situation of Mary Mallon, however, indicated something new and different. No one in the Warren household had been sick with typhoid prior to the outbreak – nor had anyone, from what Soper could discern, been in contact with anyone actively ill with the disease. To Soper's excitement, he now found himself confronted by what looked to be a 'carrier', a seemingly healthy individual who caused others to become ill.

Carriers were a very hot concept in the new world of epidemiology, a theory unproven in the United States. In Germany, however, the respected bacteriologist Dr. Robert Koch had recently investigated repeated outbreaks of typhoid in a Strasbourg bakeshop. The bakery was clean. The water supply was uncorrupted. Yet well-heeled customers were getting sick. Dr. Koch questioned the proprietor and found that she had, years earlier, contracted typhoid, but had survived the experience and was now, seemingly, fully recovered. After testing her, Koch found that even though she was devoid of symptoms and to all outward appearances a healthy person capable of working and going about her tasks like everyone else, she was in fact still teeming with typhoid germs, exuding them through her bowel movements and spreading them with improperly cleaned hands. This was a revolutionary discovery, and news of it had found its way to New York, where it was discussed with interest. Soper had read the transcript of a speech Koch had given on the subject a couple of years previous.

Dr. Soper had learned of seemingly clean and affluent homes in Mary Mallon's past being struck with typhoid after her employment. Now he was confronted with similar circumstances in yet another place she had worked. Given that no human carrier such as Koch's bakery proprietor had ever been identified in America, Soper was suddenly very, very interested in getting his hands on the mysterious Mary Mallon.

That she was evidently not interested in being found only piqued the good doctor's interest to even greater pitch:

Where is she? Of course I did not know . . . for Mary is clever, and she hardly ever works under the same name at two different places.

At this point, Soper already seems to have formed in his mind a picture of Mary as some kind of Moriarty-esque nemesis, an elusive and crafty adversary with the answer to all his questions, but always just out of reach.

He wanted her badly. His day-to-day work, by this time, had become closer to a detective's than a microbe-hunter's, interviewing witnesses, poring over records. He felt good. He was going to make his bones with this case. He foresaw himself as the poster boy for epidemiologists and health professionals, an honored and much-sought-after speaker at all the medical societies, a hero to the afflicted, a newspaper personality, idol to generations of aspiring sanitary engineers.

Furthermore, he knew that his work was important. Typhoid was lethal and, especially in 1906 and 1907, no joke.

These were boom times. It was a new century and a new world that Soper lived in. The 1900 Chicago World's Fair had once and for all convinced Americans that they lived in a great country, a major world power, on a par – at least – with the European monarchies. Any inferiority complex New Yorkers and Americans might once have felt was rapidly disappearing in the light of an increasingly power-ful, worldwide naval presence, a national construction explosion, the emergence of a newly affluent and plea-sure-seeking middle class, the recent developments of subway systems, mass-produced automobiles, a tunnel under the Hudson River, new entertainments, libraries, an exuberantly sensationalistic press, and the warm glow of having recently drubbed the Spanish in Cuba and the Philippines. Great strides had been made in the fighting of disease and the word 'epidemic' was now an embarrass-ment to a city. An earlier epidemic of typhoid and cholera had had New York and Philadelphia pointing fingers at one another, each claiming the other was responsible for the outbreak, both mortified that something so closely associated with the squalor of the old world would be blamed on their fair metropolis.

Soper's description of an earlier experience with a typhoid epidemic gives a flavor of what a man in his position saw as his responsibility, of what he perceived himself to be up against:

I went to Ithaca in 1903 when one person in ten was sick, and one person in a hundred was dying from the disease. You have no idea of the state of mind I found the people in. They didn't know what to do; didn't know where to go; didn't know whom to suspect and whom to trust . . .

These were the stakes as Soper saw them. Confusion, suspicion, contagion, neighbor pitted against neighbor, panic in the streets, and ultimately, chaos and death.

Epidemics – especially unexplained ones – tended to bring out the worst in people, and the 'carrier' theory, however fearful its implications, was far preferable to some of the alternatives. In the past citizens thought to be contagious – particularly if they were members of the minority or underclass – had hardly been taken to the bosom of their communities. Instead the usual outcome was for mob rule to win out. It was not unheard of for those thought to be infected to be run out of town on a rail or set adrift in the Long Island Sound – often at the point of a gun – or worse still. As Soper saw it, he needed a quick and tidy solution to the Oyster Bay problem.

Looking at pictures of Soper – a serious, narrow-faced,

whippetlike man with a neat mustache and a receding hairline – one gets the impression of not so much the dogged detective he might have liked to see himself as, but of a timid, fastidious scientist, a man ensconced in reasoned practice and methodology. That he might have been racist, sexist, and far too influenced by the prejudices of his class – as has been suggested by revisionist accounts – a flawed, ambitious fellow who looked for the first likely Irish woman he could clap the manacles on – does not present itself through photography. Nor do we get much of that from his work later in life: tomes with titles such as: *The Air and Ventilation of Subways (1908), Modern Methods of Street Cleaning (1909), Further Studies of European Methods of Street Cleaning and Waste Disposal With Suggestions (1930)*, and of course, what proved his masterwork, the story for which he became best known, the pamphlet with a title like a Victorian detective story's *The Curious Case of Typhoid Mary (1939)*.

George Soper looks from his photographs not to be a nice guy. He looks like someone who was bullied in high school, a nerd, a geek, an apple-polishing dirt-wonk with an unseemly interest in filth and how to make it go away.

It was not for a good many more months, not until March of 1907, that Soper finally came face to face with Mary Mallon. It was then that reports reached him that a family on Park Avenue in New York City had been stricken with typhoid. Two cases had initially been reported. A maid was ill, and a daughter of the people who owned the house, a beautiful young woman in her twenties, was lying on her deathbed. The family were reportedly beside themselves with grief. The girl died two days later, and soon the nurse who had attended her became stricken as well.

The details of the case as they reached Soper were indeed tragic, another example of bad things happening to people to whom bad things are not supposed to happen; but what particularly excited Soper, got that Sherlock Holmes mojo working again, was the news that there was a new cook fitting the description of Mary Mallon *still* employed by the stricken family.

He gushed:

Imagine my surprise and my utter joy when I found the famous germ-carrier working as a cook in that household.

The cook in question, and indeed it was Mary Mallon, did not quite share the good doctor's enthusiasm. She showed true displeasure when Soper, who rushed over to the Park Avenue address immediately upon receiving the news, suddenly showed up at her job, accusing her in no uncertain terms of causing the typhoid which right then was draining the life from one member of her employer's family.

I though after I found her all would be easy; shortly I was to be disappointed, for having found Mary I had the

greatest difficulty arranging an interview. Finally she
agreed to talk with me, and in company with a physician
I met her outside the house.

To his dismay, Mary did not see Soper as the answer to
some long-troubling question about the series of odd and
unpleasant coincidences that had long followed her. He
stood an accuser, and she reacted thus, and her reaction
seems to have come as a complete surprise to him.

Here, at this first meeting between pursuer and pursued,
is where things began to go terribly wrong – at least for
Mary Mallon and any future she might have had. What
was said here, and *how* it was said, would set the tone for
everything that happened after.

Chapter Two

Typhoid Sucks

TYPHOID: Until the mid-nineteenth century, no one even knew what it was. All that was known for sure was that lots of people were dying from it – and had been dying from it for a long, long time.

As far back as 1607, in Jamestown, Virginia, where typhoid would retroactively be credited with wiping out 6,000 settlers, officials knew something was devastatingly wrong. But people died of so many things in those years: typhus (a different disease entirely – spread by fleas and lice), cholera, yellow fever, smallpox, measles, throat distemper, influenza, scarlet fever, as well as typhoid – most of them indistinguishable from each other in eras marked by unwashed, undernourished, maltreated, and poorly housed folks who tended to die young anyway. Against a backdrop of frequent epidemics, famines, plagues, abject poverty, and rudimentary to nonexistent health care, it is no surprise that it took so long to even give the thing a name.

But in 1880, only twenty-six years before Mary Mallon went to work in Oyster Bay for the Warren family, a man named Karl Erberth isolated the particular organism associated with typhoid fever, identified it, and allowed future doctors to at least differentiate between typhoid and all the other microbes that were likely to kill you before you hit middle age. Erberth's discovery was the first step down the road to a vaccine (as opposed to a cure).

Even so, typhoid continued to be a serious problem – not the least for the military. In the war against South Africa, Britain lost an incredible 13,000 troops to the disease, a staggering body count, especially when weighed against total battlefield losses of only 8,000.

As recently as 1948, there was virtually nothing a doctor could do against typhoid, other than put the patient to bed and hope for the best. There was by then a vaccine extant, but that was like shutting the barn door long after the mad cow had wandered off to do his business. As late as the midteens, medical practitioners were still not certain that the vaccine even worked (it did). Antibiotics had not yet been discovered. So before 1948, it must have been pretty terrifying to recognize the all-too-familiar symptoms of typhoid. And they were familiar: outbreaks in 1865 and 1885 had decimated residents of major American cities. An earlier incident, when heavy rains flooded Lake Michigan, commingling sewage with drinking water, had left an estimated 90,000 dead of cholera and typhoid, so people tended to take outbreaks very seriously. In New York State alone in 1906, there had been over 3,000 cases reported, with more than 600 fatalities.

First came a sudden and prolonged high fever – brain-boiling temperatures that could reach 104 to 105 degrees. Powerful headaches followed, accompanied by gut-roiling nausea and the disappearance of appetite. Victims often developed a bad cough, hoarseness, rampaging diarrhea or constipation. Frequently adding to their discomfort and misery were skin rashes, inflammation, and tenderness in the abdomen. Until antibiotics hit the market in the late 1940s, about 10 per cent of typhoid sufferers died from the disease. Even after antibiotics, about 1 per cent still never recovered and eventually succumbed. As late as 1997, there were 17 million cases of typhoid reported worldwide, with about 600,000 deaths resulting.

Even today, in underdeveloped countries like Vietnam and Mexico, where antibiotics at first seemed to be working wonders, 75 per cent of typhoid cases are now said to be drug-resistant.

Typhoid is an infectious disease caused by a bacillus called *salmonella typhi*. Simply put, typhoid fever is transmitted by food and water that has been contaminated with human feces or urine. Polluted water is the most common source of infection. When water from toilets and outhouses drains into water used for bathing and drinking, you start seeing cases of typhoid. Shellfish such as clams, mussels, and oysters which have been taken from contaminated beds can give you typhoid. Likewise, dairy products which have had close encounters with sewage, can be – and have been – linked with the spread of the disease.

And, of course, people can give you typhoid, as long as the bacteria exists in their systems. For most people sick with typhoid, this means that for the week prior to their being bedridden (during which time they probably have not yet been diagnosed), until about a week after, they are infectious. Many (about 10 per cent) will continue to exude bacteria in their stools for about three months, and about 2 to 5 per cent will become permanent carriers, the bacteria settling comfortably into their gallbladders and digestive tracts like rent-controlled pensioners. This last statistic is important, because the beleaguered Mary Mallon was believed to be one of these unfortunate few – a carrier for life, a one-woman bacteria manufacturing machine, an endless supply of very bad things.

If you want your city, town, or prefecture to remain free of typhoid, experts recommend that you endeavor mightily to protect and chlorinate the water supply – basically keeping it sewage-free. It is suggested that human waste be disposed of in a safe and sanitary manner and that latrines be kept fly-proof. And you don't want typhoid carriers handling your food. Particularly raw food.

In Mary's time, especially in the years she was coming up and learning her trade, indoor plumbing was a fairly recent development – and in rural areas, decidedly rare. Even the idea of bathing regularly was a new, and pretty bold, concept.

Our colonial forefathers, many of whom proudly boasted of bathing only *once a year*, must have stank like musk-oxen, and the sanitary, or more accurately, the unsanitary grooming habits of generations of Americans and Europeans explains a lot about their behavior and accouterments. (That the French would take the lead in perfume manufacture should come as no surprise.) High collars, make-up, wigs, beauty marks – many of the fashion choices of much earlier days were developed as much for fashion as to cover up dirt-streaked and smallpox-scarred necks, syphilis-ravaged faces, unspeakably greasy and unpleasant hair, and rank odor. Not too much earlier than Mary's time, the 'Sunday bath' was considered the height of sartorial extravagance, something to boast about. As the turn of the century approached, people still didn't much like to bathe. They didn't, for the most part, like water. Water, it was believed, admittedly with some reason, made you sick. It gave you typhoid, cholera, fevers – all sorts of bad and mysterious stuff. Better to grease yourself up and sew yourself into your long-johns for the winter, as many frontiersmen did, than risk getting chilled and possibly ill. Better to do your business in a chamber pot, then hurl it out the window; bury it in the garden, or in the privy. Next to the well.

In the most elemental language, to prevent typhoid, modern health care professionals strongly suggest persons who prepare food for others use scrupulous care when washing their hands after using the bathroom.

It is one thing to have typhoid bacteria wriggling around inside your alimentary canal. It is another to transfer those bacteria to another human being. Not washing your hands after a bowel movement is a good way to start. Using those same hands to prepare food which remains uncooked – like, say, salad, or peach ice cream – would be better. Who among us *really* washes their hands in such a way as to satisfy the requirements of food handling? Dr. John Marr of the New York State Health Department states flatly, 'I don't know anyone who washes their hands 100 per cent after going to the bathroom.'

If you are the kind of person for whom washing your hands after a bathroom visit is an ordeal – and you allow your fingernails to grow to fashionable length – you can look forward to a real career in disease spreading. One has only to ask a health inspector to demonstrate, for instance, the proper method of hand washing for a manicured kitchen worker, then watch the professional mime furiously the scrubbing (with brush) of the undersides of the nails, top to bottom, finishing with an impressive hands-up doctor-style flourish, to get a cold chill down your spine. You'll never eat a Caesar salad again.

Chapter Three

The Conversation

WHEN INFORMED THAT the woman he had been pursuing over the last months was indeed working only a few feet away from where he now stood in the anteway of the opulent Park Avenue home, Dr. Soper could hardly contain himself.

But his enthusiasm, his bad judgment and his zeal worked against him. His first approach was clumsy:

> *I had my first talk with Mary in the kitchen of (the) house. I suppose it was an unusual kind of interview, particularly when the place is taken into consideration. I was as diplomatic as possible, but I had to say I suspected her of making people sick and that I wanted specimens of her urine, feces and blood.*

Soper tries to make excuses for getting ahead of himself, but after all, to his mind, Mary was a killer, at least of a kind, and he felt he had no other choice but to act with dispatch.

Showing up at a cook's *place of work* and attempting to interrogate her on such a sensitive subject *in front of the other household employees* and the housemistress was probably not a good idea. Demanding samples of 'urine, feces and blood' proved hardly an ideal icebreaker when attempting dialogue, especially given the fact that he and Mary had never been formally introduced.

In any event, Mary balked in a most emphatic way at Soper's suggestion that she give up her bodily fluids.

> *She seized a carving fork and advanced in my direction. I passed rapidly down the long, narrow hall, through the tall iron gate, out through the area, and so to the sidewalk. I felt rather lucky to escape. I confessed to myself that I had made a bad start. Apparently Mary did not understand that I wanted to help her.*

Soper's own accounts, given at various times in speeches, newspaper articles, and papers published in medical journals, vary as to how much was said at this first meeting. An early telling has him resuming the discussion – presumably at fork-point – outside the house on Park Avenue.

> *She upbraided me for connecting her with outbreaks of typhoid fever in every household she had worked in . . . The circumstances connected with the case were most pathetic. In the face of all this, Mary refused to submit herself to an examination and would not divulge a single fact about her past life, her relatives, her friends, in fact, she refused to say a thing to assist me.*

In another recounting (and Soper dined out on this story quite a lot), he added that Mary denied ever having typhoid fever, asserting that she could not possibly be the cause of it – either at her current employer's home or anywhere else.

Whatever words passed between them during that initial exchange, the outcome was clear. Dr. Soper went away empty-handed, and Mary Mallon went away angry, frightened, paranoid, and suspicious.

The result of that first meeting between hunter and prey was that Mary was put on the defensive. Her hackles went up and she fully staked out her position. Not guilty. Period! To get her to climb down from that particular tree would be difficult if not impossible. Soper was disappointed. Whether he knew it or not, he'd blown it. However cognizant of his own failing as interrogator he might have been, he was also, to his discredit, personally offended. It seems to have come to him as a complete surprise that the rudely ambushed cook had responded neither favorably nor agreeably to his suggestions, and this confused Soper and made him somewhat indignant.

It mattered not that I told her if she would answer my questions and give me the specimens, I would see that she got good medical attention, in case that was called for, and without cost to her.

As a matter of fact, I did not need the specimens in order to prove that Mary was a focus of typhoid germs.

My epidemiological evidence had proved that. (!) La-
boriously, I had worked out every one of seven outbreaks
and I was positive that Mary had produced them all. I felt
a good deal of responsibility about the case.

Soper was bitter that the subject of his interest was not eager to accept his offer of free 'good medical attention'. That 'medical attention' of *any* kind might have a bad connotation for her, might have sounded attractive to her only if she deemed herself sick or was feeling physical pain (she wasn't), does not appear to have occurred to him. He came away from the encounter with his position as entrenched as Mary's. She was now, in his opinion, a 'proven menace to society'.

Under suitable conditions, Mary might precipitate a great
epidemic. You can well imagine what havoc she would
have wrought if her work had taken her to poor families,
where sanitation and cleanliness are put in the back-
ground.

Already painting himself as a savior of peoples from all walks of life – both rich and poor – Soper returned a few days later to take up where he had left off, but Mary would have none of it.

It is a measure of the completeness of her denial that she had returned to work. Many would have been in the wind after the initial encounter. But Mary continued to work at the house on Park Avenue. That her employers did not immediately throw her out into the street is curious as well, signifying great indulgence on their part – or remarkable cooking prowess on Mary's.

One night, after Mary finished work, George Soper, waiting for her in hiding, followed her through the streets, shadowing her to her destination, a seedy rooming house at Thirty-third Street and Third Avenue, under the rumbling elevated train tracks and around the corner from the Willow Tree Inn and Sig Klein's Fat Men's Shop, where she appeared to be sharing rooms with a man called Breihof.

One imagines the sanitary engineer turned private dick, lurking under the Third Avenue el, spying on Mary from the shadows as she entered the rooming house. The excitement, the thrill of the chase, of sneaking around, must have been electrifying. A far cry from gazing at bacteria under a microscope, or comparing columns of statistics.

She was spending her evenings with a disreputable looking man who had a room on the top floor and to whom she was taking food. His headquarters during the day was in a saloon on the corner.

Unsatisfied with mere surveillance, Soper enlarged his portfolio of skills by now becoming a clandestine operative, a spymaster, and an agent runner of sorts. Taking note of Breihof's affection for alcohol and his limited means, the doctor-turned-case-officer entered the saloon and befriended him, plying the man with free booze while engaging him in conversation.

I got well acquainted with him. He took me to see (his) room. I should not care to see another like it. It was a place of dirt and disorder.

There was a large dog in residence, a beast of whom, Breihof confided, Mary was quite fond. The neat doctor remained in the doorway of the tawdry walk-up apartment, unsure where, or if, he could sit down. The eager-to-please, vulnerable Breihof stood there uncomfortably, revealing to the outsider his pathetic kingdom.

Breihof had turned. He'd been bought for the price of a few drinks. He cannot have been entirely comfortable with that. It was a poignant moment, for Mr. Breihof is the only known love in Mary's life. We do not know if she was ever married. We know nothing of her early experiences with men, or with love, or even her feelings about men in general. Though she was a church-going Irish Catholic woman living in less-than-enlightened times, she seems to have been living comfortably in sin with the unimpressive Mr. Breihof. It is known that later in her life, she used his name – or variants of it like Bresof (as an alias), identifying herself in some way as his de facto wife. More than likely, it was she who paid the rent on the

Thirty-third Street rooms – as Breihof had no visible means of support. And she appears to have loved him, looked after him, forgiven him his weakness for drink, and his less-than-rock-solid loyalty.

As Soper later reported.

I made an arrangement with Mary's friend to meet her in this room; and taking an old assistant, Dr. B. Raymond Hoobler, later head of the Children's Hospital in Detroit, I waited one evening for Mary at the top of the stairs.

How did he know when she was due to arrive? Because Breihof had set her up. Probably in exchange for money or drink or both.

Soper continues:

Mary was angry at the unexpected sight of me, and although I recited some well-considered speeches committed to memory in advance to make sure she understood what I meant, and that I meant her no harm, I could do nothing with her.

She denied she knew anything about typhoid. She had never had it nor produced it. There had been no more typhoid where she was than anywhere else.

There was typhoid fever everywhere. Nobody had ever accused her of causing any cases or had any occasion to do so. Such a thing had never been heard of. She was in perfect health and there was no sign or symptom of any disease about her. And she would not allow anybody to accuse her. Again I saw I was making no headway, so Doctor Hoobler and I left, followed by a volley of imprecations from the head of the stairs.

Already a fiercely private person, Mary was mortified at this latest intrusion. Her horror and embarrassment at finding Soper and associate, with their insinuations and accusations, at Breihof's door must have been shattering.

Mary knew a few things with terrible certainty at this point. She knew how serious Soper was – the degree of trouble she was in – and the apparent inescapability of it. He'd identified her secret companion, been inside her squalid little love-nest or refuge, unmasked her – surely to *his* satisfaction – as a common slut. This could only have been a hideous affront. This man, who wasn't a medical doctor but let her believe that he was, continued to insist that she was dirty, unclean, sick (a charge that can only have been bolstered by Breihof's maddeningly unclean personal habits). It was one of many humiliations to come. Worst of all, this charlatan had gotten her man to betray her, to set her up, to talk about her behind her back and allow the loathsome Soper into the room. It was an awful betrayal – and that the hapless and hopeless Breihof remained her friend and ally after this incident can only have reinforced her assessment of his weakness and her hatred of Soper for exploiting it.

For his part, Soper had, once again, proven his ineptness. What Dr. Hoobler could have been expected to add to the situation is dubious. Did Soper actually expect his doctor friend to be able to take samples from Mary right then and there? Perhaps. More likely, he brought Hoobler along for reasons of personal security. Safety in numbers. He was scared, and the thought of confronting the fearsome Mary on the landing of the cheap rooming house all by himself filled him with dread.

Notice too that Soper says he memorized his lines in preparation for the encounter, before lying in wait for her. Picture him: lying awake at night, running through the possible outcomes in his head, over and over, his palms sweating at the thought of a pissed-off two-hundred-pound Mary Mallon disemboweling him with a meat fork, that horrible dog from the apartment tearing at his groin with its hungry maw.

When Soper described Mary later as 'athletic' with 'a good figure . . . at the height of her physical and mental faculties . . . [a woman who] prided herself on her strength and endurance and at that time, and for many years after, never spared herself the exercise of it', he sounds like a frightened man, a man making excuses for being physically intimidated by a woman, a man who smells the punk inside himself. Soper comforted himself with later intimations that Mary wasn't *really* a woman anyway – certainly not a proper one:

Nothing was so distinctive about Mary as her walk,
unless it was her mind. The two, her walk and mind,
shared a peculiar communion. Those who knew her best
said Mary not only walked more like a man than a
woman, but also that her mind had a distinctly masculine
character.

It was after this incident at Breihof and Mary's apartment
that Soper finally realized his shortcomings as detective and
spymaster. Frightened, frustrated, and well aware by now
that he was unsuited to a late career change to professional
wrestling or saloon bouncing, he did what any self-respect-
ing bureaucrat would – particularly one with no powers of
arrest and no jurisdiction in the case. He passed the buck,
kicked the problem over to city officials. He raised the
alarm, went straight to the commissioner of the New York
City Health Department, and recommended that Mary
Mallon immediately be taken into custody.

I called Mary a living human culture tube and chronic
typhoid germ producer. I said she was a proved menace to
the community. It was impossible to deal with her in a
reasonable and peaceful way, and if the Department
meant to examine her, it must be prepared to use force
and plenty of it.

Soper was pleased with himself. There is an under-
current of almost hysterical glee in his descriptions of

Mary as a menacing and infectious brute – as if by calling her dangerous and unstable he was mitigating his own failure and fears.

The Department acted favorably on my recommendation. It would get the specimens peacefully, if possible, but if this was not possible, it would get them anyway.

But Soper was in fact disappointed with the initial, measured, official reaction. Rather than call out the National Guard and bludgeon Mary into submission as he might well have liked, the Health Department reacted at this point with remarkable restraint and sensitivity. They sent a woman doctor (still a fairly rare commodity in those days), the soon-to-be esteemed Dr. Josephine Baker, to see Mary at her place of work. They can be forgiven for not taking Soper's warnings as seriously as he might have liked. Perhaps they recognized his unreliability on matters unconcerned with straight epidemiology, waterborne human waste, and street cleaning. They were neither impressed with Soper's newfound identity as sleuth, nor with his unofficial standing, nor with his apparent inability to get a few samples off this Mallon person. They sent a lone woman – a qualified doctor – to the Park Avenue home where Mary was *still*, incredibly, performing her daily routines.

Soper recounts Dr. Baker's first encounter with the elusive cook, his tale permeated with a strong whiff of I-told-you-so:

The success of this gentle yet redoubtable warrior (Baker) was at first no greater than mine had been. Mary slammed the door in her face.

But the next day, to his great satisfaction, Mary was finally brought down. A horse-drawn Department of Health ambulance was sent to the Park Avenue residence where Mary worked, and parked on the street directly outside. Three policemen surrounded the house, choking off possible escape routes, while Doctor Baker, accompanied by a fourth officer, rang the basement door. Mary opened it, saw who was there, and attempted to close it again, but the cop jammed a foot inside.

The chase was on.

Mary bolted for her kitchen and disappeared. Dr. Baker and the policeman followed in hot pursuit, but couldn't find her. She was gone. The other servants clammed up, suddenly gone deaf and dumb. Baker and the police searched the basement, the closets, the coal bins, and the living quarters and came up with nothing.

Gazing out the kitchen window, Dr. Baker noticed a chair leaning against a high fence separating the house from the property next door. There was snow on the ground, and hurried-looking footprints led from the house directly to the chair and disappeared at the fence. Dr. Baker and her police escort went to the next house over, on the other side of the fence, and made a thorough search inside and out. Still nothing. They continued

44

searching for three hours, calling in yet another cop from the neighborhood for reinforcement. Again, to no avail.

Eventually, the search party became frustrated and was about to call it a day when one of them noticed a small bit of gingham caught in the door frame of an outside water closet in the backyard of a neighboring house. Ashcans were piled against the door from the outside (suggesting the involvement of a third party). They pried open the door and found Mary Mallon inside, finally cornered.

But Mary was not done. She would not go quietly. In Dr. Baker's words:

She fought and struggled and cursed. I tried to explain to her that I only wanted the specimens and that then she could go back home. She again refused and I told the policemen to pick her up and put her in the ambulance. This we did, and the ride down to the hospital was quite a wild one.

Baker describes Mary:

. . . springing from her lair – fighting and cursing, both of which she could do with appalling efficiency and vigor.

It took, in the end, five strong New York City policeman – and Dr. Baker – to subdue her.

'I sat on her all the way to the hospital,' said Dr. Baker. This episode is rife with delightful images: Fortyish

Mary Mallon, leaping out a window, scaling a high fence, and concealing herself in a snow-covered privy for over three hours in the middle of a police manhunt, an unidentified accomplice helping to conceal her by stacking the trashcans against the door. Mary, in high-necked uniform, apron and skirts, duking it out with five tough, red-faced coppers – and making a damn good show of it – all the while spouting an impressive barrage of very unladylike obscenities. Mary, struggling and flopping like a decked swordfish in the back of the horse-drawn ambulance, the relatively petite Dr. Josephine Baker sitting on top of her, as it careened down the streets and around corners on the way to the hospital.

And it's hard to decide who to like *more*: The fearsome, determined and defiant Mary Mallon, or the feisty and unintimidated Dr. Josephine Baker.

Dr. Baker would go on to become an important figure in New York State's health services, specializing in the living conditions and care of children and pregnant women. Mary's fate was decidedly less glamorous. But for a few brief moments, in the back of that ambulance, two truly remarkable women were locked in physical conflict, the pioneering woman doctor grimly following her instructions – doing a job her male counterpart had been unable to do – and an Irish immigrant woman, fighting for her life.

Mary Mallon soon found herself a prisoner, locked away in a stark white room at the Willard Parker Hospital, regarded by Soper and others as a 'dangerous and unreliable' person, who 'might try and escape if given the chance.'

So Soper states:

The room in which she found herself was in no way an attractive or particularly comfortable one, and there was no reason why a strong, active woman of forty, feeling herself to be in perfect health, should be contented with it.

And Mary was not.

Her minders were Dr. Robert Wilson and Dr. William Park, the chiefs of bacteriological labs for the New York City Health Department, and they finally, after some waiting, got what they wanted in what must have been yet another humiliating moment for Mary.

The first analyses of Mary's stool samples revealed a 'pure culture of typhoid'.

She was now thoroughly and profoundly screwed.

Chapter Four

The New Woman

It sat there, it walked and talked and ate and drank, and listened and danced to music, and otherwise reveled and roamed, and bought and sold, and came and went there, all on its own splendid terms and with an encompassing material splendor, a wealth and variety of constituted picture and background, that might well feed it with the finest illusions about itself. It paraded through the halls and saloons in which art and history, in masquerading dress, muffled almost to suffocation as in the gold brocade of their pretended majesties and their conciliatory graces, stood smirking on its passage with the last cynicism of hypocrisy.

It was the end of 1904, the beginning of 1905, and sixty-one-year-old author Henry James, touring the gold-brocaded sitting rooms and lobbies of the Waldorf Astoria, didn't much like what he was seeing. The world was changing – most noticeably in New York – and James watched in horror as the new middle class preened and played, and went about its pleasures. James's sensibilities, influenced by the more clearly delineated class boundaries of rural England, were offended, it seems, at being unable to distinguish wealthy professional from roué aristocrat, cash-flushed tradesman from blue-blooded remittance man, rich banker from rich wanker. He sounds even more bitter about the women he observed:

I . . . should not have known, at the given turn, whether I was engulfed, for instance, in the vente de charite *of the theatrical profession, and the onset of persuasive peddling actresses, or in the annual tea party of German lady-patronesses (of I know not what) . . .*

No surprise that Henry James would find all these working-class yobs with money offensive. He'd been having a bad time of it in general since arriving in New York. The subway had just been completed. Electric streetcars and elevated trains clogged the avenues. Horses, though still around, were on their way out and the newly mass-produced motorcar was on the way in. Buildings were going up everywhere, too big and too tall for Mr. James's tastes. Everyone everywhere seemed to be having way too good a time and spending too much money. This was okay in upper-class circles in England – when it was just a bunch of inbred, jug-eared, chinless aristos having their bottoms whacked and running around in top hats. But in America, everyone seemed to be getting in on the act. James didn't like it.

American observers too, particularly male ones, were unsettled by the rapid social changes going on around them. Newspaper stories of the time took delight in the cries of moral outrage issuing from the pulpit and from social commentators, and on no subject were the shrieks of discomfort and outrage more strident than when decrying the emergence of a phenomenon referred to as the 'new woman'.

> *New Woman an Abomination – She Destroys the Possibility of Being a Lover, says the Reverend W. Bruner!*

The dyspeptic reverend goes on in the text below to break down the 'problem' into three subgroups:

> *The first is the woman with children, a husband and a home, who neglects all three of them for the sake of the club, the drawing-room and the 'Temples of Pleasure.' The second class is that of women, single or married, who neglects her home duties to emphasize to the world 'women's rights'. This type is a distinct menace to society . . . The third type is the abomination of the 'childless wife'. She is too often seen in the well-fed, tastefully gowned and handsomely brought up dame who cannot bear the burden of looking after children, as such an occupation would interfere with her 'own privileges'.*

Middle-class women, like everybody else, were redefining their roles in society, redefining themselves – and having too good a time doing it for the reverend's taste. Quiet, demure, compliant women – whose sole purpose in life had previously been to get married and raise kids and run a household for their husbands, however brutish those husbands might have been, were being replaced by brainy, assertive, cigarette-smoking, self-indulgent 'new women', for whom the twentieth century promised new pleasures and real choices.

Another newspaper article of the day tried to make sense of this strange and terrible trend with the help of the Hungarian historian Emil Reich, who sorted things out for his readers thusly:

The new woman . . . is neither new nor a woman . . . In America, woman commands man and man does not count there. She lives so that she can have a good time; she lives for sensations . . . The American woman's interest does not lie in the man; she wants to be alone, and she can't be alone without dabbling, today in chemistry, to-morrow in physiology and the day after in Buddhism.

They might even start *thinking*, Reich seems to be worrying, before shifting, creepily, into some really bizarre reverie:

But she is very beautiful. She has the best complexion in the world, better than any European woman. She is well built and handsome . . . She doesn't try to have dignity or refinement. She wants to affect men by what she says, not what she doesn't say. She has no passion or sentiment, they are alien to her. She is a mass of nervous energy.

Another incensed man of the cloth, the Reverend Dr. Madison Peters, from the Church of the Epiphany, seems, like Henry James, to have found time to wander over to the Satanic halls and anterooms of Hell at the Waldorf Astoria, where he observes:

. . . nine women out of ten will order drinks of the same kind that their escorts order, and quite as many of them. I have watched these women and I have wondered if they realized what these same men thought of them deep down in their hearts . . . This brings naturally to mind the thought of why there are in this city today thousands of men in their thirties and forties, men of means or excellent salaries and incomes, who are not married. And why are there so many instances of men marrying, as society puts it, 'beneath them'?

The answer is because so many of the daughters of their own fashionable set are given to drink, cigarette smoking, gambling (for that is what bridge whist has resolved itself unto) and to kindred vices. It is because men of the world and of society realize that such women are not fit to become the mothers of their children – not fit

to preside at their table and over their household . . .
finding the women of their own circle given over to these
vicious habits, (they) go 'beneath it' and find honest
young women, whose names are not in the social
register, as their help-meets.

This sounds like positive social change, right? Anything the revs are against is surely a good thing. Fine-looking women, smoking and drinking and gambling and doing whatever they like? Sounds good! A few years earlier, women were not even given credit for being bad. Prostitutes were referred to as 'fallen' women, victims of 'white slavery', as if any independent thought – particularly when it came to matters of the flesh – was beyond their ability. Now, 'bad' women were everywhere, tearing at the very fabric of society, their most important responsibility to the world – to 'keep a good household' passed along to even more menacing and incomprehensible creatures, the servant girls.

The Reverend Doctor continues his complaint:

These women seldom read; they have no thirst for
knowledge: they seldom cultivate their minds by study.
Only the other day I was going up in the elevator of one
of the most fashionable hotels of the city when I heard a
young woman say to another, and it was then five o'
clock: 'I haven't done a thing all day but play bridge.'
That is only an example . . . the gambling whist habit

*has become so prevalent that women – dozens of them –
go from house to house, from fashionable hotel to hotel
day after day and night after night, reviving themselves by
drinks of various sorts.*

The Reverend Doctor was right about one thing.
Middle-class women were, to a great extent, abandoning
the day-to-day tasks of running a household, turning
instead into *another* kind of 'new woman', an entire
population of females for whom home, marriage, and
children had long since been discarded as the only reason
to be.

But did this amount to social revolution?

To track the true causes and effects, the factors that
really changed the lives, futures and aspirations of generations of women, you have to go back a few years, to
Ireland, to that old standard – when you're talking about
earth-shaking, population-displacing sea-change – to the
real cause of real disruption in the world order, and what
were considered to be women's roles. The true instigator
of social revolution was starvation.

Not having anything to eat makes you think. It makes
you move. It makes you do things which only a short time
earlier, you might never have considered doing. When
the food ran out in Ireland during the great famine of the
1850s, the Western world *really* began to change. Ireland
changed. It became emptier. The trajectory of millions of
women's lives altered drastically and abruptly as they

hurried to flee appallingly hardscrabble existences and probable extinction. And America, when they arrived, changed with them.

We don't know much about Mary Mallon's life prior to her first arrest and incarceration. She didn't like to talk about it – and she didn't publicly or in writings that we know of. But if you examine the history of Ireland and the Irish people in the years prior to and following her birth and her arrival in America, an illuminating context reveals itself. When we hear of Mary vaulting fences, smacking around cops, shacking up in a one-room tenement apartment with an alcoholic gentleman to whom she was not married, it's helpful to put that seemingly unique assertiveness in its proper perspective. If there were 'new women', really, in 1907, then you could hardly find a better example than Mary Mallon, a single, childless, domestic laborer pinned to the floor of a careening Health Department ambulance.

Unless you count the woman sitting on top of her, the other side of the equation.

Josephine Baker was an educated professional, a woman of some advantage who, rather than spending her time playing bridge or swanning about town imitating wealthier doyens of the upper classes, became a pioneer, dedicating her life to the field of preventive health care for children. After a private school education, when Vassar proved out of reach, she attended the Women's Medical College of the New York Infirmary, interned at the New England Hospital for Women and eventually moved from private practice to a distinguished career in public service. She lectured, authored books and was elected president of the Babies Welfare Association. As early as 1908, she was the leader of a team of nurses who taught hygiene and disease prevention in the worst districts of the Lower East Side, her efforts resulting in a significant drop in infant mortality. She was one of many remarkable women from relatively comfortable backgrounds who broke all the rules, fought the good fight, tried actively to make the world a better place – usually in the face of hostility and ignorance.

Between 1845 and 1849, four years of relentless blight on the Irish potato crop, at least a million Irish people passed away, most the victims of starvation and disease. Three million others were left absolutely destitute. Their heartless English overlords did nothing to help. As the 1851 census of Ireland puts it:

> . . . *the once proverbial gaiety and lightness of the peasant people seemed to have vanished completely, and village merriment or marriage festival was no longer heard or even seen.*

Marriage, even in furiously Catholic Ireland, was suddenly a very bad idea. If you were a dirt-poor potato farmer and your potatoes weren't coming in, taking on a wife, much less a family, didn't make much financial sense. It meant that you'd more than likely starve sooner, rather than later. Any already remote chances of moving up in the world – even in pre-famine Ireland – were diminished by the prospect of a wife and family to feed. People became reluctant to marry early – it made no sense, and parents became less inclined to subdivide their already near-worthless property holdings among heirs, as was the custom.

Irish men and women lived very separate lives. Schools were segregated. Saloons and pubs were the exclusive preserves of men and whatever limited social activity revolved around them. Disapproving clergy and relatives were everywhere, and much of male social activity revolved around drinking. Marriage, increasingly, became based on economic circumstances – and those circumstances were bad and getting worse.

From the mid-nineteenth century, the marriage rate among rural Irish declined dramatically – as did the number of children born, whether within wedlock or out of it. People were getting married less, and even when they did marry, women worked. They'd been running households for years, of course – seeing to the finances, cooking, cleaning, weaving, and in general, doing all those things which men couldn't, or more accurately, wouldn't, do. But the harsh realities of an economy based on the cultivation of the now-unreliable potato crop, required that women also work in the fields, digging turf, tending to chickens, selling crops at market. At the end of the day, the husband could go blow off steam at the pub, buy his mates some drinks, shoot a few darts, get stuttering drunk. The wife was left at home. Married couples rarely even ate together. The wife ate alone or with the children, then prepared a meal when hubby staggered home from the pub. As both parties were usually illiterate – or damn close to it – there wasn't much to talk about in front of the fire. The thought of taking the wife out for a nice walk, maybe a visit to town, did not occur to too many husbands, who felt such a display would in some way diminish them. In short, marriage, particularly for a woman, was about as much fun as a lingering illness. If she wanted something for herself, or wanted to alter her circumstances, she stood up for herself, often physically, not infrequently using a blunt object as a persuader.

With the famine, when millions of Irish peasants began pouring into New York, most of them were women. More to the point, they were women for whom the idea of deferring or avoiding marriage for economic reasons was nothing new. And they were women who were used to the idea that if one wanted to survive, one did for oneself. Men were as likely to be liabilities as assets.

Few Irish women coming to America between 1849 and 1900 came with any ill-formed intentions of 'finding a man'. They came looking to work hard, save money – and then hold on to that money. That so many of them became domestic servants who lived in the homes they served only reinforced this trend away from continued subserviency to a husband.

They were truly a self-sufficient lot, these new women, oblivious – even contemptuous – of the idea of traditional women's roles. They were proud, strong and in possession of great mental toughness. They came to America and took the work that was available – as servants and cooks to the middle and upper classes. There was a lot of work available, at least in the beginning, when almost every household, it seemed, had at least one servant. While millions of Irish women were deciding – or being forced by circumstances – to work their way into financial independence, American women, particularly of the Victorian age, struggled with the 'servant problem'. The American 'new woman' was encouraged to keep a good house, but without getting her hands dirty. Her responsibility was to 'educate' her servants in the proper skills and comportment required of a 'decent household'. The servant and the cook became, in this atmosphere, an essential, if frequently joked about, element of middle-class life, and they damn well knew how indispensable they were.

By 1900 most Irish domestic help had had about enough of being looked down on and maltreated, and were having no more of it. Negotiations over working conditions and wages were often contentious. Any misguided attempts to legislate propriety amongst one's servants in their leisure hours often resulted in frustration. Domestics, after working all day and into the evening, having no families to care for, and limited funds, often spent their off-hours in activities deemed inappropriate by their mistresses. Hanging out in saloons, buying dresses too similar in style to their mistresses' than their mistresses appreciated. With a few bucks in their pockets and a nice dress or two, the unattached, unsupervised domestic servant girl could hang out in the beer gardens and dance halls, Bowery clubs or bars – maybe even enjoy a little slap and tickle.

Employment agencies for domestics became prime recruiting grounds for whoremasters and brothel owners. Women heads of households were urged to take the training of their servants as a religious calling – the 'spiritual' benefits of appropriate behavior being thought as important as their cooking and cleaning skills. It's hard to believe they persevered against such independent and determined subjects. How do you instruct a woman who's already survived incredible hardship, who's worked hard all her life, on how to live 'properly', when your life is, by contrast, a carefree wonderland of excess, sloth and caprice? When many families found it difficult to afford the number of servants they felt they required, attempts were made to form food 'co-ops', central associations where family meals could be prepared in a central location and delivered, cost-effectively, to households. This development did not go over well with traditional domestic cooks – and many of them organized against the co-ops, blacklisting families who had engaged their services, even threatening to go on strike. Families who underpaid or mistreated their help would find themselves infamous in the increasingly vibrant and vocal subculture of domestics, and such organized schemes such as price fixing and standardization of practices and working conditions were enacted, however informally, by networks of working women who exchanged information, resolved disputes, debated what tasks they could and should be responsible for in a given situation.

These women became an important segment of the New York City economy. They saved when everyone else seemed to be doing nothing but spending. Between 1819 and 1847, early years yet for Irish immigration, domestic women servants accounted for almost two-thirds of all savings accounts opened at the New York Bank for Savings.

What you had, by Mary's time, were large numbers of women who were used to standing up for themselves, who determined, to a greater degree than almost any other group of women, their own destiny, who were resourceful, having to contend with employment situations where they often bounced from one job to another. (Summers were particularly difficult. Many families ran off to Long Island and Maine for vacation. Mary Mallon's steady employment during these times speaks well of her skills as cook.) These were tough women, unused to taking guff from anyone. Accounts of the day on the subject of stubborn and belligerent servants were legion – the stuff of popular jokes and anecdotes. Lydia Marie Child, quoted in Marie Stansell's *City of Women*, describes an Irish domestic confronting a gentleman on the street who has ordered her summarily out of his way:

> '*And indade I won't get out of your way; I'll get right IN your way!*' . . . *She placed her feet apart, set her elbows akimbo, and stood as firmly as a provoked donkey.*

Stansell goes on to describe a few saltier phrases, quoting from court depositions of the time – all with Irish female defendants:

> *She would 'knock her brains out' . . . 'tear his guts out'.*

Sound familiar?

Mary Mallon was one of *these* new women. Formed out of poverty and abuse, newly arrived in a strange land, where the Irish were, for some time, considered only slightly elevated from apes. They were 'white niggers', without a pot to piss in, and as women even less likely to raise themselves from their circumstances. Without family or husbands, they learned to hustle, to negotiate, to endure. They acquired marketable skills and demanded to be paid for them. It was from the early practices of avoiding marriage, working for themselves, saving money, learning, that Irish women began moving into professions like teaching and nursing. At a time when most professions were considered unsuitable for women, many began to break through.

Their examples did not go unnoticed. The children of the rich, inspired, perhaps by their parents' Irish help, began misbehaving.

A news story from 1906:

RICH WELLESLEY GIRL WAITRESS IN HOTEL
She is nineteen and the daughter of Alfred E. Bosworth,
a wealthy banker . . . (she) acquired democratic ideas of
life through associations with another girl who earned her
college expenses during the summer by serving as a
waitress in a hotel and she decided on the same course
herself. While other girls were leaving for the seashore or
foreign countries, Miss Bosworth, in a plain white
dress . . . had secured a position in the dining room
of the Mount Pleasant House in Breton Woods.

Or this one from the same year:

VASSAR GIRL IS REAL CINDERELLA
Preferring to work as a servant girl rather than marry the
man she did not love, Katherine Gray, a Vassar grad-
uate, and the daughter of the late Senator Asbury Gray
of Virginia . . . has been employed as a house servant.

'He was old enough to be my father,' said Miss Gray.
'And I told Uncle so: but he insisted, and finally told me
that if I did not marry the Major, I must leave the house.'
Miss Gray took the latter alternative.

Mary Mallon was not a revolutionary. But she was part of a revolution. She wasn't that different from hundreds of thousands of other women who'd been cut loose from one oppressive system to make her way in another. She was unluckier than most – in that she was *identified* as carrying typhoid. But like many of her peers, she was a fighter, a scrounger, a hustler, and a hater. She wanted her piece of the American Dream and was all too willing to work for it. They just wouldn't let her. She did the best she could.

Chapter Five

The Cook's Lament

MAYBE, if some strange kercheifed man with a big, gold hoop earring had whispered out from a Hester Street storefront, ' Mary! There's a hoodoo following you!' then she would have believed it. She had to know something wasn't right. A curse? A hex? Evil spirits?

It was true that the sickness – 'typhoid' – seemed to follow her. She couldn't argue with that. She'd seen it firsthand. She'd even stayed on at the one home – the one in Maine – to nurse those afflicted, so she'd seen it up close. She'd seen the fever and had an idea how it must have felt and knew that *she* didn't have *that*. *She* was healthy as a horse.

Sickness was everywhere. People of *her* station were always getting sick, dying. Down at the saloon where Breihof liked to drink, they had a term for it, 'getting your elevens up'. One of the regulars – some hard-drinking old geezer – would disappear for a few weeks and then reappear, looking dissipated, the cords on the back of his neck deeper and more pronounced, the two muscles jutting straight up from the man's collar like two 1's. The others at the bar would wait until he was gone or out of earshot and simply shake their heads slightly, mutter

65

'Looks like so and so's got his elevens up' – meaning the poor bastard would be dead soon enough.

Death and disease and starvation had been nipping at her heels from the beginning. Back in Ireland, it was the way of life, they died by the thousands, the exact cause – if ever identified – simply a postscript to the inevitable. People died in their beds. They died in the fields. They were lucky if they didn't die in their cribs.

Mary was born in Cookstown, County Tyrone, Ireland, in 1869. About fifteen years later, like so many of her starving countrymen, she fled to the United States, penniless, in steerage, aboard a sorry, crowded packet. They died on the boat too. She'd been watching people die her whole life, in increments. One day sick. The next? Gone. For her, life had *always* been an endless vista of suffering and struggle. She knew about epidemics. The world was *full* of them!

From 1873 through 1875, it was influenza – swept through Europe and America like the four horsemen. In 1878, in New Orleans, the last great wave of yellow fever . . . in 1895 it was Plymouth – typhoid this time (Was *that* her fault too?) . . . in Jacksonville, Florida, there was yellow fever again, though not as bad as New Orleans . . . and later, much later, there would be more: a worldwide influenza epidemic would wipe out more people than were wounded in the Great War. U.S. Army training camps would become giant sickwards, with an 80 per cent fatality rate.

Some people got sick. Some died. Maybe God decided. Who knew? Mary had felt herself lucky – as if, perhaps, someone was looking after her – as if there *were* rewards for her hard work and her sacrifices. She'd stayed single, childless. She'd kept herself up. She'd prayed. She'd tried to lead a decent life – unlike so many others of her country and profession. They said – the doctors and the engineers and the health department coppers – that dirt had something to do with it; they were always going on about washing your hands and such. But Mary knew what dirt was. She'd seen *real* filth and *she* certainly wasn't dirty like that. Nowhere near. She kept herself *up*, her apron clean, her uniform always white and ironed. It was the weak that got sick. Then they got sicker. Then they died. It was always like that, wasn't it? How could they say she had the fever? *She* certainly wasn't weak. No one could say that about her. It was a point of honor how strong she was, how fit.

And here's this man, this miserable interloper, minding everybody's business but his own, claiming to be a doctor (she had her suspicions) – a man who doesn't even know her – who doesn't know how *strong* she is, saying she's dirty, sick, a menace to others. What did he – in his nice suit and his carefully trimmed mustache and his prissy manner –know about sickness? Poor people were always sick. That's what the poor *did* – they got sick and died, usually in droves. The people down the street when she first came to America, the people down the hall, the crowd at Thirty-third and Third – one day they were there, the next in a box, family and friends crowded around the coffin in a tiny tenement living room. 'Old John? You didn't hear? He's passed. Gone. The wake was last week. Lovely spread they laid out. Terrible thing.' Back in Ireland? It wouldn't have even been 'Old' John – it would have been, 'Didja hear about young Johnny? His mother was in here today. Terrible thing. Terrible. Two little ones out of four . . .'

Who noticed *them*? No one in *this* city. Certainly not if it were Irish doing the dying. The good citizens of New York were too busy, everyone rushing about in their new automobiles, digging holes in the ground, putting up buildings so tall they were an offense to God almighty, putting on airs, dressing up, always hurrying off someplace. The upper classes? The rich? The new trash who'd suddenly come into money and liked to rub your nose into it? They didn't care. They didn't notice. Until one of their own goes ill. Then it's a sodding emergency. Some privileged prat starts feeling poorly and then it's call out the Marines, start looking for someone to blame – a hardworking, decent Irish woman, for instance.

Before, they had said it was the water that did it. It was settled. The typhoid came from the water, they'd said. That time in Tuxedo Park? They said then it was that laundress who brought it into the house, brought it in with the washing. And who could be surprised at that?

The woman had looked sick from the first! Anyone could see. Stuck out a mile.

Why were they picking on her? Why Mary Mallon?

Someone must have said something. Another servant more than likely. It was jealousy, plain and simple. The servants, the laundresses, they always resented her. Didn't much like emptying out the coal from her oven. Didn't care to do the washing up either – and did a damn pitiful job of it most times too. Mary had a skill, a talent. That made her special; it brought her a little extra. And of course, in the kitchen, she was the boss. The rest never liked that either. They didn't like it when she upbraided them for messing with her things, pilfering the food, sticking their dirty fingers in the ice cream.

These health officials called *her* dirty? They should have a good look at some of the dirty birds sticking their dirty paws into her food when they thought she wasn't looking.

What to do now? The job? That was gone. She could kiss that off. The agencies were put wise – tipped off by that meddling Dr. Soapbox. They wouldn't be sending any work her way any time soon. Even if she got out. Not ever. References? Might as well drape herself in the skull and crossbones.

What next? Who'd hire her?

Now they were calling her a killer – a murderess. They didn't exactly put it that way – not quite. But that's what they were saying – once you got past all that silky double-talk and fake cheer. Once *that* got around, she was properly buggered. They'd said they'd keep her name a secret, but who could believe anything they said?

She carried the sickness inside her body, they said. She spread it with her dirty hands. Who could believe such things? She'd never felt better in her life!

If she was so sick, how come it had taken five policemen to subdue her? Could a sick person do that? Could a sick person jump out a window, climb a high fence, then wrestle five policemen to the ground and curse the lot of them?

It was persecution, simple as that.

It was *their* rotten lot that was sick. *They* were the ones obsessed by shit and piss and indecent things – the ones who wanted to put the knife on her, cut out her gall-bladder. They wanted to know about her family, her friends. What she got up to with any gentlemen. So they could spread their lies. Nosy Parkers. More than likely they'd like to track *them* down as well, maybe lock *them* up. No trial. No judge. One day safe in her kitchen – the next, locked up in solitary confinement: white room, white bed, white sheets, white robe. Questions every day. Strangers come to gape. And more questions.

She wasn't going to tell them anything.

Not a fucking word.

Chapter Six

A Good, Plain Cook

COULD MARY MALLON COOK? If she walked into your kitchen right now could she whip up a nice meal from available ingredients?

The best indicator that Mary Mallon *could* cook well is her employment history. Even with an incomplete record, it's clear that between 1900 and 1906, Mary was employed fairly steadily by well-to-do families, even during the summer months, when many domestic cooks struggled to find employment as their patrons deserted Manhattan for vacations on Long Island, Maine, and New Jersey. It's hard to believe that Mary was what we call today a 'ham and egger,' a utility cook with a limited repertoire of lumbering Anglo/Irish standards and little else. The requirements of the time were demanding. Mary had a lot of competition. When she first came to the attention of authorities, the city and the country were in the middle of a foodie boom.

They even had a name for these food-crazed gourmands – this vanguard of foodie nouveau riche: 'Lobster Palace Society' – a floating demimonde of the sort later referred to as 'Café Society,' folks like Oscar Hammerstein, the boxer Gentleman Jim Corbett, the architect (and later murder victim) Stanford White, Bet-a-Million Gates, Diamond Jim Brady and his frequent companion, Lillian Russell. In 'Lobster Palace Society,' where everyone, it seemed, was encouraged to outdo one another in the new pastime of conspicuous consumption, the female icon, the desirable template for female beauty, was the decidedly hefty Russell, who weighed in at a porky 230 pounds. Though famed for her colossal eating and drinking binges, this hardly detracted from Russell's popularity or perceived beauty – if anything, it enhanced it. Popular objects of desire of the day were Lydia Thompson's 'British Blondes', women who looked like the defensive line of the Pittsburgh Steelers. In his book *On the Town in New York*, Michael Batterberry tells us that the portly poster girls would keep 'in shape' by wolfing down 'midnight suppers of anchovies on toast, sirloin steak and potatoes, tripe and onions and wedges of Stilton'. It was not only okay to get fat, it was fashionable. Men's clubs threw gigantic 'Beefsteaks', orgies of overconsumption which could last all day and into the night, marathons of steak and chop eating and oyster slurping accompanied by gallons of beer. More relevant to Mary Mallon's day-to-day life, excesses in style were all the rage; service and servicewear could be elaborate, with theme nights being particularly popular. Evenings at Delmonico's, Rector's, and Sherry's were marked by such innovations as meals served and eaten on horseback, parties where gigantic pools were erected so that food could float by on miniature re-creations of guests' yachts, dinner parties for dogs. At more notorious events, strippers bathed themselves in champagne and emerged naked from cakes. No outrageous indulgence seemed too much.

The pressure was on. French chefs were enjoying special popularity, and poor 'Brigit', the fabled and much-reviled servant girl, was under pressure to compete – or at least emulate their examples. Hosting evenings, teas and dinner parties was the ticket to social status for the new rich. One can only imagine Mary's torment when her latest mistress read about some Turkish-themed party in the society pages and demanded Mary learn 'the cuisine of the Orient'. Cookbooks and fad diets and manuals on housekeeping and proper deployment and use of domestic help were all the rage. It must have been a challenge. A new 'movement' seemed to pop up every day, preaching on one hand simplicity, and on the other excess and extravagance. The public, it was said, was eating too much protein, not enough grain, too few vegetables. There were too many domestics, not enough of them. Poor Mary must have wanted to strangle her employers at least once a week. Kitchens were beset by new developments in technology, sanitation, with an influx of new, absolutely necessary gadgets being advertised and endorsed almost every day. Charles Ranhofer's groundbreaking book *The Epicurean* had allowed every housewife with reading skills to think she could re-create previously out-of-reach French classics. Even the cookbooks and manuals advocating simple, time-saving recipes read like the instructions for a missile launch or complicated neurosurgery.

You might think that turn of the century diners were used to limited variety, clumsy and unsophisticated fare. You'd be wrong. Menus of the day offered raw shellfish, offal, French classics – alongside German and English/American stand-bys. Things like jellied pig's knuckle sat alongside turkey wings à l'Italienne and risotto. Luchow's on Fourteenth Street offered ragout fin en coquille, beef goulash with spaetzle, calf's head en tortue. The Rorer Restaurant, a fairly prole establishment by comparison, offered three types of oysters, New England clam chowder, relishes, fried soft-shell crabs, hard crabs, fried chicken Maryland, broiled bluefish, baked whitefish au gratin, sandwiches of tongue, sardine, roast beef, corned beef, turkey, lobster and caviar! The Ladies Lunch at the Metropolitan Club featured such carnivore-friendly offerings as deviled kidneys, kidneys en brochette, mutton chops, curry of chicken livers, broiled sweetbreads jardiniere, roast squab, smoked tongue. Reiseweber's on Columbus Circle, billed as an 'Electric Grill and Gentleman's Club and Bar', served up a menu of seven sweetbread entrees, thirteen chicken dishes, fifteen potato sides, and a huge assortment of desserts, ice creams, fruits, brandied fruits and cheeses. The fish section alone contained sea bass, mackerel, sole, bluefish, halibut, salmon, frogs' legs, and lobster. The Breslin, after a course of oysters or clams on the halfshell, saucisson de Lyon, caviar, and vermicelli soup, might offer a fish course of butterfish sauté meuniere, followed by cold dishes like galantine of capon, gumbo strained in jelly, terrine de foie gras Strasbourg, pâté of game, fricandeau of veal with parsnips.

Fancier menus, created almost exclusively by French and European chefs, set the tone for second-tier, dazzling with an incredible array of continental piece montées, tallow carvings, pastry displays, ice carvings, ingredients like snipe, thrushes, woodcock, robins, preparations which paid homage to faraway lands and exotic cuisines – like turbot vol au vents, timbales of pike, chaydfroids of larks, bouche à la reigne, paupiettes of fowl, gratin of eel, fried brains, Nesselrode pudding, roebuck filets with noodles, crab cakes, coulibiac – this was pretty intensive stuff, a lot of which (the coulibiac for instance) would make any modern-day cook, with all his Cuisinarts and Hobart mixers and blending wands and paco-jets, blanche with fear.

This was not simple food being dangled in front of the eager noses of the new and eager middle class. Some of it – in whatever form – must have trickled down. Mary's employers were unlikely to settle for their guests being served beef and potatoes or typical 'English/Irish' cuisine. Not every day, anyway. No way. At the very least, if Mary wasn't reading the latest recipes, it's likely she had to be able to follow them when the boss came over, head filled with croquembouches and vol-au-vents. She had to know what she was doing.

Matters were made less agreeable by the fact that the prevailing cuisine was European – with French being preeminent. The mantra of *all* French chefs and the first principle of *all* French cooking is, of course, to 'use everything.' One didn't simply bone out a chicken, serve the nice white, skinless breast for dinner, then discard the rest – or feed it to kitty – as more modern and lazy generations of Americans did. When one served steak, in a restaurant or at home, the mark of a good and frugal cook was to find ways to use the rest of the animal – or whatever parts were at hand. French cuisine is great for exactly this urgent need to find ways to make the tough and unlovely bits attractive and delicious. Shanks and shoulders must be braised slowly, tongues, kidneys, hearts, tails, lungs, hooves, and snouts used whenever possible. Innovative but often difficult, time-consuming and pains-taking procedures and recipes were developed to accomplish that end. Chefs became great chefs because they knew how to use every scrap, coax every bit of flavor and substance out of every bone, scrap and trimming in order to make money for their masters while still dazzling their customers. French cuisine grew up around this grim duty to make fiendishly clever use of everything that swam, crawled, slunk or pushed its way through turf. Look at some French 'classics': coq au vin (tough, over-exercised bird, slow-braised in red wine until tender – often thick-ened with blood), tête de veau (gelatinous, rolled-up face and skin of veal, stewed until tender) perhaps accompanied by sauce ravigotte (leftover egg yolks from meringue, emulsified with oil and garnishes), pieds cochon (pigs' feet, bones torturously removed, stewed, reassembled, baked en gratin with mustard and bread crumbs, i.e., stale bread), boeuf bourguignonne (tough hunks of fatty shoulder meat, stewed until tender), tallow sculptures (discarded beef fat), escargots (nasty snails disguised with garlic butter). Even the vaunted Delmonico's – which offered over a hundred different soups on any given day – played the game, operating within this kind of crafty/ frugal mindset: throw a little of yesterday's tomato soup together with today's pea soup, and you have potage 'mongole' – three soups for the price of two! Keeping up with the Joneses, in Mary's time, required serious knife skills and a fairly comprehensive knowledge of how to butcher, merchandise, and coax various critters into ed-ibility. Baking, pickles, preserves, the making of ice creams, cakes, cookies, were bottom-line skills, funda-mentals in even the simplest of households. Add the food craze of those kooky, crazy times to the mix and you have – at best – one serious pain in the rear end for even the most accommodating domestic cook in the home of a member of the new rich.

It might have been easier for an Irish cook – in a time when one seldom got two weeks' notice and unemploy-ment benefits did not exist – to continue pleasing one's cruel masters with the simple standards of English/Amer-ican workhorse dishes if they never entertained and if the cook also performed household duties. Many, if not most, homes had exactly that kind of arrangement. But Mary, notably, worked in larger households, where chamber-maid duties, maintenance, laundry, and so on were taken care of by other servants. Mary got jobs and held them on the basis of cooking – and cooking alone. More was expected in such a situation. Both family and their guests, presumably, had to be dazzled – and this was increasingly difficult to do in a cash-rich, food-crazed world where everybody was not only eating, but reading about eating, rushing to restaurants and hotels and dinner parties and clubs. And this was – remember – New York!

As technology improved, Harvey Levenstein points out in *Revolution of the Table*, the middle classes used their kitchens and dining rooms to improve their social stand-ing. If one's cook was not exactly Escoffier, at least one could bury one's guests in exotic ingredients. Even cook-books and menus which appealed to Anglo-American practitioners, aimed at middle-class homes, suggested menus like this one from Maria Parloa:

Oysters on the halfshell followed by consommé à la royale . . . followed by baked fish with hollandaise . . . cheese soufflé . . . roast chicken with mashed potatoes, green peas and cranberry jelly . . . oyster patties . . . salad with French dressing . . . cheese and crackers . . . frozen pudding with apricot sauce, sherbet, meringue, sponge cake, fruit and coffee.

Assuming Mary had to make anything like this, one must also keep in mind that she had already served the family breakfast, lunch, and maybe even afternoon tea. Even assuming that Mary was indeed a 'good, plain cook' with a repertoire of Anglo-Irish classics, it cannot have been an easy life. In smaller homes, in the early part of her career, and in later, harder times, it is likely that she shared in some laundry chores. Mary, it was said, was an excellent seamstress – particularly talented at crochet work. So surely she had experience there.

We know for certain that she was very good at ice cream. Peach ice cream in particular was well remembered – even by her victims. Sadly, it was exactly this specialty that was the probable source of transmission for many of her victims. As Soper correctly points out, cooked food, by the time it reached its cooking temperature, would have killed any typhoid germs Mary might have transferred. Ice cream and raw peaches, however, would have been a very attractive medium. The relatively high number of fellow servants afflicted suggests that chambermaids and laundresses, passing through Mary's kitchen, might have grabbed a piece of raw fruit, nicked a raw string bean, stuck a finger in a tub of ice cream on occasion – which would explain their higher rate of infection.

The turn of the century marked an explosion in prepared and prepackaged foods, taking *some* of the heat off the beleaguered cooks of the day. You could now have bread, meat, fish and the like prepared for you and delivered to the door. Baking powder had begun being added to flour, making leavening a lot easier. Canned soups and vegetables, cereals and mixes were advertised on attractive little picture cards which were distributed door to door by salesmen, soon to be replaced by even more popular magazines filled with ads for all the absolutely new necessary gadgets. Kitchen designs became simpler and more sensible, with easy cleaning in mind, and we can safely assume that by 1907, at least in the wealthier homes where Mary worked, she enjoyed all the modern conveniences: nonporous congoleum floors, tin ceilings, ceramic-lined two-chamber pot sinks, the latest in zinc-lined iceboxes – and most importantly, a gas stove. This last development, which appeared in the late 1870's and early 1880's, was a marvel and widely in use by the turn of the century, particularly in the homes of the rich in urban centers. While Mary had certainly learned to cook on the massive, sooty coal- and wood-burning stoves of yesteryear, it's likely that by 1907, she was well accustomed to the modern convenience of a cooler-burning, cleaner, and easier-to-use gas stove – with its easy-access water heater (for hot water washing). Ingeniously designed cabinets and work stations had become popular, usually sporting a fold-down work area with storage for tools and dry ingredients above and below. This was all wonderful– but it must have made it difficult on some of her summer jobs – and later wilderness years – when she worked for less affluent households and had to go back to hauling coal.

Cleanliness – a concept which Mary had been accused of ignoring – was hardly foreign to her. Sanitation was a mania in kitchens of her time. Carbolic, ammonia, alcohol and soap were as much a part of domestic cooking as meat or vegetables. Housekeepers were urged to practice monthly or at least seasonal cleaning, in which absolutely everything was stripped down, hand scrubbed, dusted and polished like on a navy vessel. Ceilings, floors, walls, moldings, the insides of drawers, tops of pipes – the insides and outsides of all appliances, the garrets, pantries, stairs, every single utensil, plate, glass, curtain, carpet, ottoman, gee-gaw and pillow had to be washed thoroughly. The two-chamber pot-sink, much like the sinks of our time, was kept filled with scaldingly hot water for cleaning and rinsing and polishing of flatware and dishes and the battle against dirt and contagion were hotly discussed and debated issues in home manuals and magazines and books. Yet Mary suggested, through her lawyer, that some of the kitchens she'd worked in where typhoid later appeared were not the cleanest, most well-appointed facilities in the world. No snob like a working-class snob. A coal stove, in a summer home in 1906, might have been an irritant to a domestic cook used to Park Avenue opulence.

Cooks who arrive to find an old dirty kitchen, ignored by generations of their predecessors, rarely improve the situation once it has been left to fester. They find it hard to resist the concept of 'It was like that when I found it'. If the pots and pans in a kitchen are encrusted in years of baked-on carbon, most cooks shrink from chipping and scraping them down to their original luster – and in kitchens where pockets of filth and grease have been allowed to collect, they will often sweep and scrub around them. It's a phenomenon any chef is well aware of – which is why so many are fanatical about every tiny detail. One slightly carbonized pot becomes the harbinger of general disorderliness, and each stain, each neglected accumulation of dirt is seen as a clarion call for the forces of chaos and filth.

It has been said that Mary was not particularly fastidious. Was that hindsight – a conveniently comfortable retroactive musing from those left at the scene after the ambulances and hearses had departed?

What is clear is that the equipment, the mindset, and the personnel there all suggest an atmosphere of careful food handling. It's not like the idea of washing your hands after visiting the bathroom was some goofy new theory. People were busily tearing up old floors and putting down tiles, ripping out wainscoting and filigree, doing away with curtains, putting up easy-to-wipe tin ceilings . . . stripping down their kitchens to make them cleaner, lighter, easier to work in – all in the name of cleanliness. Mary was probably dunking her hands in searingly hot water, ammonia and carbolic all the time. She wasn't a stupid woman. What was *wrong* with her?

Chapter Seven

Exile Near Main Street

WITH MARY SAFELY RESTRAINED at the Willard Parker Hospital, Dr. Soper felt more comfortable about paying her a visit. The first time he dropped by, he found her 'curiously healthy' and, unsurprisingly, 'fearfully angry looking'.

> *'Mary', I said, 'I've come to talk with you and see if between us we cannot get you out of here. When I have asked you to help me before, you have refused, and when others have asked you, you have refused them also. You should not be where you are now if you had not been so obstinate. So throw off your wrong-headed ideas and be reasonable. Nobody wants to harm you.'*

When this speech made no impression on her, Soper continued:

> *'You say you have never caused a case of typhoid, but I know you have done so. Nobody thinks you have done it personally. But you have done it just the same. Many people have been made sick and have suffered a great deal; some have died. You refused to give specimens that*

would help to clear up the trouble. So you were arrested and brought here and the specimens taken in spite of your resistance. They proved what I charged. Now you must surely see how mistaken you were. Don't you acknowledge it?'

Mary just stared back silently ('gleaming angrily') at the sanitary engineer.

'Well', I continued, 'I will tell you how you do it. When you go to the toilet, the germs that grow within your body get upon your fingers, and when you handle food in cooking they get on the food. People who eat this food swallow the germs and get sick. If you wash your hands after leaving the toilet and before cooking, there might be no trouble. You don't keep your hands clean enough.'

Mary continued giving him the blank stare, but Soper persisted.

'The germs are probably growing in your gallbladder. The best way to get rid of them is to get rid of the gallbladder. You don't need a gallbladder any more than you need an appendix. There are so many people living without them.'

Mary's eyes, according to Soper, widened slightly at this point.

'Mary', I continued, 'I don't know how long the Department of Health intends to keep you here. I believe that depends partly on you. I can help you. If you will answer my questions, I will do everything I possibly can to get you out. I will do more than you think. I will write a book about your case. I will not mention your real name; I will carefully hide your identity. I will guarantee that you will get all the profits. It will be easy for you to answer my questions. You know what I want to find out Above all, I want to know if and when you have had typhoid fever, and how many outbreaks and cases you have seen.'

Maybe a white-on-white cell was not the best environment to pitch Mary on a book deal. Especially when the proposed literary project involved discussion of her toilet practices, her habit of infecting people with typhoid and causing them to die, and the removal of her gallbladder. No small amount of self-incrimination would be required – and what decent person would want to read such a book? Maybe he should have taken her out to Rectors or Sherry's before launching into his book proposal, showed her some nice cover art sketches – ones that made her look good. Surely that was, even then, the accepted approach. It's hard to believe that even an unemployed carnival freak, Jo-Jo, The Dog-Faced Boy, for instance, would have looked kindly on such a deal under such circumstances, without even a free lunch and more seductive surroundings to help things go down easier.

Mary wasn't interested in any damn book.

[She] rose. She pulled her bathrobe about her and, not taking her eyes off of mine, slowly opened the door of her toilet and vanished within. The door slammed . . . It was apparent that Mary did not intend to speak to me.

North Brother Island is a twenty-acre knob of glacial detritus which pokes out of the East River about twenty-five hundred feet west of Rikers Island. It's just east of the Port Morris section of the Bronx, where the river takes a turn towards the Long Island Sound and the currents are nasty. Claimed by the Dutch West India Company in 1614, North Brother and its smaller sibling, South Brother, about five hundred feet southeast, were referred to as 'The Companions' until 1695, when the British government granted them to a Mr. James Graham. The two islands were left uninhabited for nearly two hundred years. In 1871, North Brother was sold to the town of Morrisania in the Bronx, which also did nothing with the space – surrounded as it was with treacherous waters. A lighthouse keeper and family were apparently the only residents until 1880.

In 1860, New York City's population had soared to 813,669 people, an increasing percentage of that number consisting of Irish immigrants. Many of them were sick.

Many of them were unruly. It's fair to say that the wealthy and powerful men who ran things in those days weren't too happy about all these foreigners pouring onto their shores and were eager for someplace to put them. Space was needed to put away the infected and infectious, the felonious, the indigent and the strange – preferably someplace where New York's solid citizens wouldn't have to see them. 'Hulks', or prison ships, had been used during the Revolutionary War – but with hideous results, so the government couldn't simply float society's undesirables offshore, say just over the horizon. Unused and unattractive pieces of real estate in the middle of the East River were the next best thing, it was thought, and first Blackwell's Island, then Randall's, Ward's, Hart, North Brother, Rikers, and Ellis were being used to warehouse the unlovely. There is some reason to believe that these islands were *already* being used as a de facto refuge for typhoid, typhus and TB sufferers who'd been shunned or driven away by their neighbors.

North Brother Island first hosted a hospital and tent city for the Sisters of Charity to house typhus patients, but there was a more pressing need. Residents of small towns in Westchester were chasing smallpox victims into the city, unwilling and unable to take care of them themselves. Through various maneuvers of arm-twisting and ward-heeling, it appears, the city convinced the suburbs to build their own facility – a shack on the East River where they could pen up their sick. Unfortunately, when residents found that the one patient at the new place was black, they mobbed the place, set it on fire, and chased the patient and caretaker onto a boat. The two washed up on North Brother Island and squatted in an existing cottage.

In 1885, perhaps inspired by this example, the city built Riverside Hospital. They built it in a hurry, as there was a typhus epidemic going strong and it was anticipated that they would soon need the room. Staten Island wouldn't play ball – the citizens of that island didn't want any hospital filled with contagion carriers on *their* island. The other islands in the East River were already building other facilities, and the city had even had to *build* two islands (Hoffman and Swinburne) to keep up with demand for space. North Brother seemed the perfect out-of-sight, out-of mind place in which to quarantine the herds of typhus, cholera, yellow fever, and smallpox victims overflowing from other facilities. In 1898, the hospital began to be used primarily for Bronx residents – with exceptions made for matters of urgent need.

It was ugly. It looked, from above, like a ramshackle Alcatraz: At the outset, a two-story brick building for eighty patients, with three frame structures for forty each for busy times. It wasn't enough. By 1900, tuberculosis was everywhere, killing thousands, and in 1903, two new buildings were erected and even that wasn't enough. Over the next few years they continued building – the city even had to pour landfill into the river to make room for even more structures. If you were poor and talked with an accent and were unlucky enough to get tuberculosis, you might well find yourself at Riverside Hospital on North Brother Island.

North Brother was not a happy place. In 1904, three years before Mary Mallon was exiled there, the island was the site of its most notable tragedy; the fire on the 264-foot *General Slocum* excursion steamer. A witless deckhand had been careless with straw and on June 15, the second-worst fire in maritime history broke out in the storeroom, ultimately causing the deaths of 1,021 members of the German community who'd chartered the vessel to take them to Huntington, Long Island, for their seventeenth-anniversary picnic. Most of the passengers drowned, dragged down by faulty or fraudulent life preservers. Lifeboats were unusable or nailed to the decks, the firehoses rotted, and the captain, apparently, oblivious until it was too late. The ship in flames, with passengers falling and leaping into the current, the captain headed ashore at North Brother, the ship's movement only fanning the flames and accelerating the destruction. Residents of the Bronx and New York paddled out to the scene in any available vessels, primarily to rob floundering Germans and to strip the dead. The living, still struggling in the rough water, were largely left to drown, or extorted for money before being rescued. More helpful were some prisoners from nearby Rikers Island, who actually swam over to help before returning to their cells. The charred and drowned bodies of 611 dead Germans were soon laid out in a row on the lawns of North Brother Island, with another 400 still bobbing in the river.

It was not an island with a happy history or an attractive present. It was about as far away from the world as a place could be and still be in New York. This was where Mary Mallon was banished in 1907. She was housed in a small bungalow which had once been home to the head of Riverside Hospital's nursing department. It was situated at the southern end of the island and contained a living room, kitchen and bathroom and all the conveniences of the time: gas, electric and modern plumbing. It was, as Soper overgenerously describes it, 'pleasantly situated on the river bank, next to the church.'

Her food was brought to her. She prepared it and ate it alone. Across the water she could see the city.

She was now serving an indefinite term of confinement. She had never been charged, indicted, tried, or convicted of any crime. Her face was in the newspapers; a sketch artist had come to Willard Parker and captured her image. The press had begun calling her 'Typhoid Mary'. She was famous.

Chapter Eight

A Typical Cook

'*She is a large, healthy-looking woman, a typical cook, and there is nothing in her outward appearance to indicate that she is other than normal. She is, of course, segregated with the typhoid patients.*'

So said Dr. William H. Park of the Board of Health. The statement was erroneous. Mary, at the time, was the lone typhoid patient on the island.

When we consider that she has been spreading the contagion for years, it is clear that she will be a prisoner on North Brother Island for a long time, perhaps for life; certainly until the (typhoid) germs and (typhoid) tendencies have been eliminated from her body.

Every effort has been made by the health authorities to cure the unfortunate woman, but so far without success. Examination is made each day with the hope that some one of the various expedients we have tried may put an end to the discharge of bacilli. Nothing we have tried so far has proved effective.

There is a later photograph of Mary at North Brother Island, huddled in a blanket among a row of similarly swaddled typhoid patients on the 'sunny side' of the pavilion. It looks like Stalag 17. The women sit close together as if sharing warmth. Their backs rest against a plain wooden wall, their feet on haphazardly lain-down planks to keep them out of the mud. What 'expedients' the doctors were trying on her to, as one paper put it, 'dry up the fountainhead of typhoid germs in Mary Mallon', is anybody's guess. Medical literature of the time does not inspire confidence – nor can Mary's limited experience with doctors so far have reflected well on the profession. She was a new phenomenon in the annals of typhoid. Doctors came to chat. They came to gawk. They came to suggest new treatments. And she listened to what the doctors and the nurses said, hanging, as patients do, on every word, analyzing the differences between their various recommendations, looking to glean something hopeful from the contradictions. The constant refrain continued to be the suggestion that she have her gallbladder removed. Would this cure the problem? No one could say with any assurance. It just seemed like a good idea, something they'd like to try – the preferred option from what must have seemed to Mary to be particularly unsympathetic, bumbling, and knife-happy jailers. She was not, it can also be said, popular with the other patients.

She was a cook. Who saw herself, as many cooks do, as

slightly better than everybody else. Not higher on the evolutionary scale, nor better in the social sense of the word. Just harder-working, more skillful, more righteous. And she was, after all, a martyr of sorts. Identified in the press as the notorious Typhoid Mary, she was the subject of ribbing and gossip and speculation. She had little else to do with her time but stare out at the river, watch the world going on without her and recount the outrages committed against her good name and person. She had a lot of time to think – and was aggrieved and angry, and she did what any modern-day citizen with a gripe would do: she got herself a lawyer.

How Counselor George Francis O'Neill became involved in the case is unclear. He was a shrewd choice. Twice a Republican candidate for the state senate, prominent in Irish affairs, he had been, prior to taking the bar exam, a customs inspector, a man well versed in public health issues. There have been suggestions that the hidden hand of William Randolph Hearst is visible at this point in the story of Mary Mallon. Hearst, not unlike the quasi-portrait of him in the film *Citizen Kane*, had swept back into town by storm in 1895. In 1887, after a short stint working at *The New York World*, young William had convinced his dad, George, to buy him the *San Francisco Examiner*. When George kicked off in 1891, he left 17 million bucks to his wife, William's mother, and William, already jacked on newspapers, immediately hit mom up for some dough – wanting desperately to return to

New York and carve himself out some territory in the highly competitive newspaper business. Obligingly, mom sold off 7.5 million dollars worth of Anaconda Copper shares and gave the proceeds to her son. For the bargain price of 180,000 dollars, William Randolph Hearst bought himself the *Morning Journal* in 1895.

The early episodes of *Citizen Kane*, in spirit at least, portray pretty closely the real-life Hearst's stint in New York. He wanted things. A lot of things. Among them was to be president of the United States. He set himself up as the advocate for the working man, the underdog, the downtrodden and the unfortunate, railing (at times fearlessly) against Tammany Hall politicians, social injustices, corruption, and inequity as he saw it. And he behaved, in public at least, with rectitude – never swearing, avoiding alcohol and tobacco.

There was one principal obstacle, however, one other pretender to the throne of Spokesperson for the Masses and Champion of Virtue; Joseph Pulitzer, whose own newspaper, the *World*, proudly crowed that *it* was the champion of the downtrodden. Hearst quickly began an energetic, no-holds-barred circulation war between his paper and Pulitzer's, positioning himself, unashamedly, as the voice of the nation. His involvement in Cuban exile politics and his fomenting of war with Spain is well known. He was not, for instance, beyond fabricating alleged Spanish atrocities. Even Pulitzer saw a war with Spain as too good to miss out on and joined the fray, only ratcheting up the stakes. In the end, Hearst spent 7 million dollars trying to knock his rival out of the game, lavishing money on foreign correspondents, cables, and innumerable extra editions, most of which were returned for rebates. But in the end, both papers ended up with a circulation of about a million and a quarter. Hearst's *Journal* swallowed up the *World* and William got at least most of what he wanted, a loud and influential voice, a presence in national journalism and politics – and he used both assets with vigor.

He was sympathetic to the Irish, certainly. This was both tactically wise and seemingly heartfelt. Any imagined constituency would be largely Irish working class and have to, by necessity, include and appeal to the large numbers of public servants, politicians, Irish organization members, eating clubs and wardheelers who made the day-to-day of New York politics run smoothly and profitably. An editorial in the *Journal-American* on St. Patrick's Day reveals a near-militant admiration for the cause of Irish republicanism and goes on to excoriate Americans for their relative gutlessness and compliance in the face of adversity and inequity.

And *Journal-American* coverage of the Mallon case was relatively restrained – even actively empathetic.

Did Hearst hire George O'Neill for Mary? Did Hearst see a continuing legal battle – pitting a hardworking Irish woman on one hand, and the monolithic Health Department with all their loosely defined powers to incarcerate and evict and restrain on the other – as a good thing for circulation? *Somebody* was being awfully nice. Or was it O'Neill himself – working pro bono perhaps? Hearst had provided lawyers for subjects of articles before – or helped organize fundraising for legal defense – and the Hearst papers' coverage and access could certainly indicate a closeness to the case which other papers seem not to have enjoyed. *Someone* was paying for the services of the Ferguson labs.

In any case, Mary Mallon found herself with a distinguished advocate. Over the next few years, while she never *won* a motion or a case, she clearly either wore the opposition down or, at the very least, scared them mightily.

After two years on North Brother Island, Mary Mallon, with George Francis O'Neill at her side, appeared before Justice Erlanger, claiming that there was no law on the books to justify her continued detention. By now, June 29, 1909, there had been a few developments in her favor: fifty additional persons had been identified as typhoid carriers in New York State alone and yet none of them had been confined to North Brother Island or to jail. The 'health menace' she had represented two years earlier had faded somewhat in the public's memory.

The spin on the news story had changed. Even some of her jailers began to sound sympathetic and troubled by the implications of her case.

Chapter Nine

Habeas Corpus

THERE'S A FINGERPRINT SMUDGE on the handwritten affidavit of Mary Mallon aka Typhoid Mary, dated April 12, 1909, where she seems to have attempted to rub away an extra consonant in the word 'anything'. The penmanship is excellent – classic Palmer method, with nice loops and valleys – and the spacing is neat, for the first few pages. But as the impassioned, and at times angry account proceeds, the writing gets sloppier, the text takes on a downhill slant, the content becomes less diplomatic. It's a fascinating peek inside the head of a very angry cook and it's almost all we've got to remember her by. In her answer to the affidavit of Dr. Park of the Board of Health, Mary speaks in her own words:

I am not segregated with the typhoid patients . . . there is nobody on this island that has typhoid . . . there was never any effort by the Board authorities to do anything for me excepting to cash [sic] me on the island and keep me a prisoner without being sick nor needing medical treatment . . . when I first came here [Mary did not bother with punctuation or caps – unless referring to names and titles] *. . . they took two blood cultures and* *feces . . . [then] three times a week say Monday Wednesday and Friday respectfully until the latter part of June . . . after that they only got the feces once a week which was on Wednesday . . . now they have given me a record for nearly a year for three times a week(!!)*

Mary is here referring to a document submitted by the Corporation Counsel, representing the Department of Health in response to a writ of habeas corpus from her lawyer, O'Neill. The paper chronicles the 'bacteriological results of the examination of feces from Mary Mallon' from dates beginning March 20, 1907 and ending June 16, 1909. And she's half-right: scrupulous, three-time-a-week sampling continues until December of 1907, at which time things change – from three times a week to five times a month, then four times a month, sometimes three. It must have been puzzling, even suspicious, to Mary, who, like any patient who has heard troubling news, was looking for reason – any reason – to hope. Maddening also were the results. 'No typhoid found' for weeks in a row, followed by 'typhoid found' for a few days, followed by 'no typhoid found' and back again. Her friend Breihof, apparently, had been forgiven for his snitching, and remained devoted. He now shuttled Mary's stool samples to the privately engaged Ferguson Laboratory for analysis in the hope of disputing the Department's data – and there do appear to have been incongruities. The Ferguson results, without exception, found no typhoid, perhaps because Ferguson was telling the client what they wanted to hear, or maybe because Breihof was not conveying the samples in a timely fashion and they had degraded, perhaps while he enjoyed a few libations. Mary, at least, seems to have put some stock in them. The court did not.

This part of the story is troubling because at this point, Mary seems to have begun to put stock in *somebody's* laboratory analysis. She is no longer sweepingly condemning *all* medical science – particularly when they're telling her what she wants to hear. She's selectively believing what *some* doctors and nurses are telling her – lifting bits of what they've said and what she's overheard, and winnowing out that which she sees as useful to her case.

'When I first came here I was so nervous and almost prostrated with grief and trouble my eyes began to twitch and the left eye lid became Paralyzed . . . remained in that condition for six months . . . there was an eye Specialist visited the Island three or four times a week and he was never asked to visit me I did not even get a cover for my eye . . . had to hold my hand on it whilst going about at night . . . when Dr. Wilson took charge he came to me and I told him about it . . . he said that was news to him and that he would send me his electrick [sic] battery he never did such . . . However my eye got better thanks to the Almighty God and no thanks . . .

Here she thinks better of what she was about to write, and scratches out the 'and no thanks.'

The affidavit moves on to describe some of the medical 'expedients' and 'strategies' her warders have been using to rid Mary's system of typhoid.

In spite of the medical staff Dr. Wilson ordered me Urotropin . . . I got that on and off for a year . . . sometimes he had it and sometimes he did not . . . . I took Urotropin for about 3 months all told during the whole year . . . if I should have continued it would certainly have killed me for it was very Severe. Every one knows who is acquainted in any kind of medicine what what it's used for Kidney trouble?

Mary, evidently, was listening to the nurses, comparing what the various doctors told her, and forming her own opinions about treatment. She had, a year before filing her habeas corpus, engaged another lab to do their own testing – and she had willingly provided samples for them. She was becoming something of a jailhouse doctor and the seemingly haphazard testing, treatments and results were obviously frustrating and provocative – suggestive of sinister motives and incompetence. What O'Neill and Breihof were telling her, culled from their own information gathering efforts, and what she had gleaned from her limited contacts on North Brother, must have offered maddening little anomalies and rays of hope which she clung to fiercely, believing those things which might reflect positively and rejecting the negative.

When in January they were about to discharge me when the resident Physician came to me and asked me where I was going when I got out of here . . . naturally I said to NY . . . so there was a stop put to my getting out of here . . . the supervising nurse told me I was a hopeless case and if I'd write to Dr. Darlington and tell him I'd go to my Sisters in Connecticut. Now I have no sister in that state or any other in the US . . .

Were the doctors and Health Department functionaries of the State of New York trying to unload the Mary Mallon problem on another state? The head nurse seemed to be doing just that. All Mary Mallon had to do was lie – tell them that she was *not* going to remain a New York problem – that she was going off to live with a notional sister out of state. It's a telling detail that she refused to play ball here. And that rather than take that offer and play that game, she instead, rather stubbornly, used this episode as evidence of duplicity in her affidavit.

Then in April a friend [surely Breihof] went to Dr. Darlington and asked him where I was to go away . . . he replied that woman is all right now and she is a very Expensive woman but I cannot let her go my self . . . the Board has to sit . . . come around Saturday . . . when he did Dr. Darlington told this man I've nothing more to do with this woman . . . go to Dr. Studiford . . . he went to that Doctor and he said I cannot let that woman go and all the people that she gave the typhoid fever and so many deaths occurred in the families she was with . . . Dr. Studiford said to this man go and ask Mary Mallon and inveigle her to have an operation performed to have her Gall Bladder removed.

Here Mary quotes Studiford as saying, 'She'll have the best Surgeon in town to do the cutting.'

I said no . . . no knife will be put on me . . . I've nothing the matter with my gall bladder . . . Dr. Wilson asked me the very same question I also told him no . . . then he replied it might not do any good . . . also the supervising nurse asked me to have an operation performed . . . I also told her no and she said the remark would it not be better for you to have it done than remain here . . . I told her no . . . There is a visiting Doctor who came here in October . . . he did take quite an interest in me . . . he really thought I liked it here that I did not care for my freedom . . . he asked me if I'd take some medicine if he brought it to me . . . I said I would so he brought me some Auto-Auto tox and some pills then Dr. Wilson had already ordered me Brewers Yeast . . . at first I did not take it for I'm a little afraid of the people and I have a good right for when I came to

*the Department they said they were in my tract . . . later
another said they were in the muscles of my bowels and
lately they thought of the gall bladder.*

This is not some illiterate, ignorant lumpen, oblivious
and blindly disbelieving of anything to do with modern
medicine. Mary Mallon sounds like a very angry convict,
acutely aware of the lapses and inequities of her case. She's
been informed of the progress – or lack of it – in her
treatment, appalled by the conflicting theories and opinions in her case – and underwhelmed by the level of
humanitarian concern and attention paid. She sounds
spiteful – and spite, a powerful motivator in many cooks,
explains much of what occurs later.

*I have been in fact a peep show for Everybody even the
Interns had to come to see me and ask about the facts
already known to the whole wide world . . . the Tuberculosis would say there she is the kidnapped
woman . . . Dr. Parks has even had me Illustrated in
Chicago . . . I wonder if he, Said Dr. Wm. H. Park,
would like to be insulted and put in the Journal and him
or his wife called Typhoid William Park.*

On this up note the affidavit ends. It is interesting that
Mary has chosen to be so publicly indignant. There are
indications that she had simply played the part of the
confused and helpless victim of circumstances.

O'Neill's petition to the court was more carefully worded and succinct:

> . . . Said Mary Mallon is being confined without commitment or other order of any Court within the State of New York, or that of any other person or authority having power to restrain her, in a building connected with the Riverside Hospital, North Brother Island . . .
>
> That said Mary Mallon is in perfect physical condition, and has since March 6th, 1907 the date whereon she forcibly and without warrant or order of any character [was] placed in the custody of the department of Health, never been obliged to receive the care and attention of a physician or surgeon, and that she is not in any way or any degree a menace to the community or any part thereof.

He goes on to urge the court in argument to allow Mary Mallon her immediate freedom.

> If such an act as this can be done in the case of any person said to be infected with typhoid germs, it can be perpetrated in the cases of thousands of persons in this city who might be infected with tuberculosis and other kindred diseases. If the mere statement that a person is infected with germs is sufficient then the person can be taken away from his or her home and family and locked up on North Brother Island. That is what has happened in this case.

We absolutely deny that this woman has ever suffered or is now suffering from the affliction alleged. It may be safely assumed and we have charged that in some of the households where this woman was employed the conditions were most unsatisfactory and unsanitary and the cases of typhoid referred to by the officials of the Health Department may undoubtedly be ascribed to this.

This woman has been a victim of unfortunate circumstances in having been employed in houses where typhoid broke out, the disease having been unquestionably the result of conditions which she had nothing to do with.

It's an impassioned-sounding and clever argument. It offers the artfully crafted statement that Mary was not 'suffering' from typhoid, and suggests an alternate theory of the case – and not an unreasonable one. There *were* other typhoid carriers out there. There were other causes. While the circumstantial evidence provided by Soper was compelling (the original letter drawing attention to the case was suspiciously lost) it was shaky in spots. And the prospect of *any* contagious patients being hounded – without due process – into isolation wards was a very real one.

In support of the Department of Health were affidavits from Soper and Dr. Westmoreland, the resident physician at Riverside Hospital, stating that Mary Mallon was, in fact, infected with the typhoid bacilli and that during a period of eight years she had been responsible for twenty-six known cases. Turning the knife, mention was made of the 'severe struggle' it took to apprehend her.

Press observers speculated on her fighting ability and weight class, wondering out loud how much trouble she'd be able to give the cops should they have to come for her again. She was 'rosy as you please and [looked] as though she could make . . . valid resistance'. This account goes on to describe her woefully holding a page from a Sunday newspaper. It is doubtful, judging from her affidavit, that she was happy to have her face in the papers under the header 'Typhoid Mary', but this particular journalist thought otherwise. 'She held in her pocket a page . . . a picture of Typhoid Mary dropping skulls into a skillet, Mary seemed to think that was a good picture of herself notwithstanding the sentiment.'

The usual suspects gave background interviews. One Health Department source claimed that 'if she should be set to work in a milk store tomorrow in three months she could accomplish as much as a hostile army.' A Dr. Walter O. Beusal of Bellevue refers to her as a 'great menace to public health, a danger to the community, and on that account she has been made a prisoner. In her wake are many cases of typhoid, she having disseminated – or as we might say, sprinkled – germs in various households. Mary exhales thousands of typhoid germs with every breath she expels. She has been doing this for several years, the juggler of germs say . . . a human typhoid fever factory . . .'

That typhoid fever is not generally 'sprinkled' or spread by airborne transmission seemed to matter not to Dr. Beusal. Even Dr. Park seems to have cranked up the hyperbole a bit, admitting that while many other carriers existed, Mary was 'the chief', because of her profession and her known belligerence.

Of course, O'Neill was exactly wrong. The Department of Health *did* have the power to arbitrarily lock up anyone they damn pleased. Their strange and terrible powers went further than that; Section 1170 of the Charter of Greater New York states specifically:

> *Said board may remove or cause to be removed to proper place . . . any person sick with any contagious, pestilential or infectious disease; shall have exclusive control of the hospitals for the treatment of such cases.*

Section 24, Chapter 383 of the Laws of 1903 goes further:

> *It shall require the isolation of all persons and things exposed to such diseases . . . It shall prohibit and prevent all intercourse and communication with or use of infected premises, places and things.*

Counsel refers to the legal precedent of *Seavey vs. Preble*, where the judge ruled that:

To accomplish and prevent the spread of contagious or infected disease, persons may be seized and restrained of their liberty and ordered to leave the state; private houses may be converted into hospitals and made subject to hospital regulations, buildings may be torn down; infected articles seized and destroyed, and many other things done which, under ordinary circumstances, would be considered gross outrage on the rights of persons and property . . . When the public health and human life are concerned, the law requires the highest degree of care. It will not allow of experiments to see if the less degree of care will not answer . . .

People ex rel. Lodes vs. Department of Health:

Boards of health . . . act summarily, and it has not been usual anywhere to require them to give a hearing . . . before they can exercise their jurisdiction.

The final nail was Section 42, page 102:

The danger to the public health is a sufficient ground for the exercise of police power in the restraint of liberty of such persons.

The court came down on the side of caution and established law. Justice Erlanger, on July 16, 1909, ruled that:

The risk of discharging the inmate of the Riverside Hospital is too great to be assumed by the Court. The injury which may be done to innocent persons . . . are incalculable . . . While the court deeply sympathizes with this unfortunate woman, it must protect the community against a recurrence of spreading the disease.

Justice Erlanger was, however, troubled by some aspects of the case before him. He offered that 'Every opportunity should . . . be afforded this unfortunate woman to establish, if she can, that she has been fully cured. And she may, after further examination of her . . . renew the application, or, if the petitioner prefers, the matter may be sent to a referee . . . to take testimony and report to the court with his opinion . . . This will allow her the opportunity to cross examine witnesses called against her and to offer her own medical experts to sustain her claim.'

This part of the opinion could not have brought joy to the Health department. Over the next few weeks and months, it is probable that they had to give serious consideration to how amateur sleuth George Soper would hold up under a withering cross-examination. A 'battle of the experts' is something no attorney likes to deal with, especially when the subject matter is at the very spear tip of medical theory and practice. There were documents missing. Varying and contradictory and plainly wrong-headed accounts given to newspapers. And the petitioner cut a sympathetic figure. There were troubling implications for anyone sick with a contagious illness or for anyone who was caring for a family member with such an illness. There was the Irish dimension – the Health Department *could*, without too much trouble, be portrayed as anti-Irish in its policies. All too many immigrants from all over the world had endured all sorts of outrage on Ellis Island and at the hands of the Health Police. The judge was aware of this when he ordered that Mary's living conditions on the island be 'examined and ameliorated.'

Just the same, Mary Mallon was sent back to her bungalow on North Brother Island. Angry, disappointed, and with diminished hopes for the future.

Still, she did have an admirer.

A Mr. Reuben Gray, age 28, of Lansing, Michigan, wrote the health commissioner, Dr. Thomas Darlington, suggesting a solution to everybody's problem. He urged the commissioner to pack Mary off to Michigan – 'quietly, as the Michigan health authorities might object' – so that he might make her his wife. He felt for the embattled and imprisoned Mary, he explained, adding that he himself had once been declared insane – but that he now was considered sound by 'alienists of recognized authority'. Whether Darlington passed along this proposal is unlikely.

During the whole habeas corpus episode, the press, and particularly the Hearst papers and the socialist rags remained extremely sympathetic to Mary's plight. Mary herself had suddenly become media savvy, working the civil rights angle for all it was worth. She even rather shrewdly gave an interview to Hearst's rival, the *World*. She appears to have sat for a portrait (which, by the way, made her look lovely). 'As there is a God in Heaven, I will get justice somehow', she was quoted as saying. 'She says she has been kept like a leper . . . with only a dog for company', wrote one reporter – though the evidence shows that she did have some friends and acquaintances at Riverside – and that her days were not quite the Devil's Island routine she portrayed. Mary had more for the fourth estate: 'The contention that I am a perpetual menace in the spread of typhoid germs is not true . . . My own doctors say I have no typhoid. I am an innocent human being. I have committed no crime and I am treated like an outcast – a criminal. It is unjust, outrageous, uncivilized. It seems incredible that in a Christian community a defenseless woman can be treated in this manner.' Another quote from her is near poetic in its lofty assertions:

There were two kinds of justice in America . . . All the water in the world wouldn't clear me from this charge, in the eyes of the Health Department. They want to make a showing; they want to get credit for protecting the rich, and I am the victim.

One Hearst reporter even suggested that the evil doctors, in Mary's mind anyway, might knock her out with ether and 'perform a surgical operation to prove their theory.'

'She became', in the words of Dr. John Marr of the New York State Health Department, looking back at the case decades later, 'a cause célèbre. She sold papers. She was a *character.*'

While the newspaper coverage of the Mallon hearing was sympathetic – and even a little intimidating to the Health Department posse – and raised issues troubling to the judge, it did not affect the result. Someone, however, seems to have been moved by newspaper accounts: In 1910 the new health commissioner, Lederle, under pressure and clearly exasperated by the whole predicament of Mary Mallon, referring to her as 'that unfortunate woman', suddenly ordered her release.

He tried to explain his unexpected action to a skeptical press:

She has been released because she has been shut up long enough to learn the precautions that she ought to take. As long as she observes them I have little fear that she will be a danger to her neighbors. The chief points that she must observe are personal cleanliness and the keeping away from the preparation of other person's [sic] food.

I have taken a personal interest in her case and am doing what I can for her. It seems to me that the people of this city ought to do something for her. She is a good cook and until her detention had always made a comfortable living. Now she is debarred from it, and I really do not know what she can do. I do know where she is but must decline to give any information on this point. She has promised to report to me regularly and not to take another position as a cook. I am going to do all I can to help her.

Lederle, aware that at least fifty other carriers had been identified statewide (with none of *them* similarly incarcerated) went on to state that others were similarly infected and suggested that growing awareness of this fact had been a factor in his decision. She had not, he admitted frankly, 'been cured'.

But she has been taught how to take care of herself. Her danger to the public was due entirely to the fact that she was a cook. She will change her vocation and will at stated intervals report to the Commissioner of Health for examination. He will at all times be appraised of her address.

A reporter inquired as to what Mary Mallon would do now.

I do not know . . . but I am trying to find some position for her. She ought to have a chance. She has in my opinion been hounded long enough for something that was no fault of her own. She was incarcerated for the public good and now it is up to the public to take care of her. There should surely be some reciprocity in this case.

When reporters pressed him further, wanting to know if *any* of the treatments tried at Riverside had even decreased the generation of typhoid bacteria in Mary's system, Lederle barked,

> *I can't say that. Her safety to the public does not lie in that. It lies in the fact that she now knows how to prevent their spread and that she will change her employment. For Heaven's sake, can't the poor creature be given a chance in life?! An opportunity to make her living and have her past forgotten? She is to blame for nothing – and look at the life she has led!*

Mary Mallon had clearly either talked at length with Lederle, or he'd followed her case closely and read her interview with the *World*; his statement is filled with images which can only have come from her tale of mistreatment and woe. The experts had not, it appears, offered a more palatable solution to the dilemma. Mary's bacteriological count had not responded to treatment. With O'Neill playing hardball on one side, and Mary playing a more compliant game on the other – at the very least nodding approval to the suggestions of careful hand-cleaning and an end to cooking as a career, Lederle had an out. He let her go, throwing her on the mercy of the public.

Now, let's be real. Nobody was going to step forward and offer Typhoid Mary a job in their hardware store or notions shop. Jobs for women, at best, were extremely limited. What, exactly, Lederle had in mind when he asked for 'reciprocity' and for the public to 'take care of her' is unknown. It is known that someone, probably the Health Department, hooked her up with a laundress job, but she thought the job beneath her.

A few months after her release it became obvious that Mary Mallon was *still* very much upset with the people she saw as having ruined her life, and that she was unimpressed by the sympathetic Lederle's efforts and statements on her behalf.

In December of 1911, she announced through her attorney that she was suing the City and Doctors Park, Westmoreland, Darlington, Soper, and *Lederle* for $50,000 in damages, claiming that because of their actions she was 'unable to follow her trade of cooking' and that her 'chances of making a living have been greatly reduced.'

O'Neill made a halfhearted pass at the court of public opinion, stating, 'If the Board of Health is going to send every cook to jail who happens to come under their designation as "germ carrier" it won't be long before we have no cooks left and the domestic problem will be further complicated. What would the poor jokesmith do then for his stories about the cook who rules the house?'

Mary had no chance, and her attorney knew it.

Spite ruled. *How* aware was Mary of the reality of her condition at this point? To what degree did she believe or suspect that the doctors and the Health Department might have been right? It didn't matter any more.

Chapter Ten

On the Lam

MARY'S LAWSUIT against her tormentors never came to trial. It is likely that her attorney, O'Neill, prevailed on her to drop it. The courts had found no difficulty depriving her of her freedom, and it was unlikely in the extreme that they would award her a quick fifty thousand for her pain and suffering.

It's not too hard to imagine how unhappy she was. After working her way up to cook, to find herself laboring as a lowly laundress must have been embittering. She had been the boss, in charge of kitchens in fine homes. Now she was just another anonymous drone, doing unskilled labor with unskilled laborers and for half the money. She'd been publicly reviled, nicknamed with an unforgettable moniker, locked up, poked, prodded, examined, interviewed, depicted in photos and illustrations, gossiped about, teased – and now was back at the bottom. Forty-one years old and a laundress in an outer borough, indistinguishable from younger, stupider, less experienced girls who might well have been just off the boat. What gets you through a soul-destroying workday in a job like that – and in such humbling, even humiliating, circumstances? Hate. Desperation. Spite. Fear. Anger. None of those are good things in a person with a potentially dangerous and infectious disease.

To make matters worse, her boyfriend, Breihof, became gravely ill. A heart problem became so bad that Mary arranged for him to be admitted to hospital. And once again, the medical profession gave Mary no reason to love it. They couldn't help her man. Breihof died in the hospital. The know-it-all doctors, the same kind who'd been so sure about Mary's condition, couldn't save her poor man. She'd stuck with him – as he'd stuck with her. She'd forgiven him his treachery with Soper. She'd overlooked his drinking and his uselessness. She'd lived in sin with him, going outside the church, setting herself apart from others and perhaps, in her mind, from God. Now he was dead. And she was alone.

What mattered now?

She was worn down. And she had nothing to lose. She stopped checking in with the Health Department, and she disappeared. She began, once more, to do the one thing she knew she was good at, the one thing she could feel a measure of pride in, the thing that brought her money and a measure of respect: She cooked.

It had to be tough. Almost all the good families in the New York area got their cooks from either of two employment agencies, Mrs. Stricker's or Mrs. Seeley's. Mary's face was, by now, thanks to Soper, well known at both. The name Mallon was certainly not a selling point. Under aliases, Mary began working again – not in the fine homes of the rich, but anywhere she could.

She drifted from job to job. Tried briefly to operate a rooming house. That didn't work out. She worked in a restaurant, Healey's on upper Broadway, in a sanitarium, an inn in Huntington, a big hotel in New Jersey. Anywhere they were willing to pay her to cook and weren't too scrupulous about her part or her name. That's one of the advantages of cooking for a living – then and now: Nobody cares where you came from.

From being the boss of the kitchen, Mary now toiled alongside other refugees and desperadoes in the hot, cavernous kitchens of hotels, restaurants, and institutions.

Soper claimed later that there were cases of typhoid reported at some of these jobs, though there was, he said, 'No record of them'. He claimed that the list of afflicted included two children – and that a man for whom Mary mixed a home remedy for indigestion was later hospitalized with typhoid. 'For five years Mary traveled about New York and its vicinity without restraint and without her identity being discovered by the authorities', Soper wrote. 'I was not asked to find her again, but I think I could have done so.'

For five years Mary bounced around, the world growing up around her. While her countrymen rose up in society, grabbing their piece of the pie, assimilated into the middle class, graduated into the power structure, Mary sank unnoticed to the bottom.

Did she know? Did she know she was spreading typhoid?

Yes, of course, she knew. Maybe she couldn't look at it. Or wouldn't look at it. But she knew. She'd thought enough of the methodology of the Health Department to engage her own laboratory. She'd provided stool samples willingly enough to *them* – regardless of the negative results. There had been the implied threat of the lawsuit. And she *had* to take note by now how people seemed to get typhoid a lot when she was around. The woman *knew*. She just didn't care. They'd taken everything from her. She had no reason to love anyone, not the doctors, not the public, not her employers, not the people for whom she now cooked.

If you think this is an unusual attitude for a cook, you've never worked a busy short-order kitchen. You've never been in the restaurant workers' union. Where cooks are anonymous, plenty gets lost in the sauce.

Hostility to the customer, towards the whole world outside the kitchen doors is not unusual. It's a tradition. There's us and those like us – no sympathy for anyone else. This is not to say that cooks in good restaurants hate their customers and are busily hocking and spitting and folding their effluent into their food. No, no, no . . . it's just that cooks, who work in isolated, hot, airless spaces, under tremendous pressure, lose perspective, they lose sight of *who* they're actually cooking for. All those bodies out there in the dining room, clamoring for food, always wanting more, more, more – the tables turning, more customers taking their places, the bottomless, gaping maw of the hungry public becomes, at times, monolithic, an abstraction. A sous-chef in a fine restaurant will spend hours preparing for service, setting up mise-en-place, conscientiously tournéeing perfectly shaped little vegetables, staggeringly beautiful garnishes, lovingly reduced sauces – finally their station is ready . . . all crocks and bins and containers are full, sauces topped off, meat portioned and positioned for easy access. Everything is perfect. Everything is in its place. The universe – as cooks know it – is in perfect order.

Then the customers come and ruin it.

The attitude in less proud and conscientious kitchens is even more adversarial. One is not likely to hear a cook say, 'Pick up that refired venison for the fine folks on table seven.' They're going to say, 'Here's the blankety-blank venison for those blankety-blanks on seven!' The party of ten in the dining room whose order is causing the whole hot-line to shut down while the cooks struggle to arrange and garnish their plates at the same time are not individuals – they're an immediate problem to be solved with cold-blooded and disembodied efficiency. When you're working in a nursing home, or a sanitarium, or institution where 'cooking' often means dumping vast buckets of gruel into steam tables, then refilling them as they run low, the relationship between the cook – all the way down in a subcellar prep kitchen – and customer becomes even more theoretical. It only gets worse if cook and customer come face to face in such circumstances. Day after day of actually *watching* people loading their trays with food you know is barely qualified to be called slop, piling on more than any will ever eat, chawing their chow with their mouths open, looking through the hapless worker, behind the counter as if they didn't exist, lining up and sliding their trays and loading their plates compliantly, like a herd of cud-chewing steer is, to know real hate, however unspecific and unfocused. When you're preparing, say, Welsh rarebit for six hundred people every day, what's a single lost Band-Aid? Who's to know – or even care – if you accidentally sneezed in the food, forgot to wash your hands, mixed the moldy cheese and the swill milk with your bare arm up to the elbow fresh from emptying your oil pan, or unclogging the grease trap?

By 1915, after five years on the lam, working under the names Brown, Breihof, and others, Mary Mallon was a pretty beaten-down cook. Whatever she might have thought of herself, whoever it was she once thought herself to be, had long since disappeared, supplanted by a string of aliases and a series of bad jobs. The small, clean, well-ordered kitchens she'd once enjoyed, the respect of her coworkers and clients, the love of a man, the food she'd once made, the typhoid she'd been accused of carrying – these had all faded into the grim, day-to-day requirements of slopping out sludge to an ever-changing and faceless horde. There was the job. And nothing else. Save bitterness.

In March of 1915, there was an outbreak of typhoid

fever at the Sloane Hospital for Women, a maternity hospital on Fifty-ninth Street and Amsterdam Avenue in Manhattan. Twenty-five people, most of them doctors and nurses, became ill. Two persons were said to have died.

Exactly what happened next is open to controversy. Here is what Soper would have us believe, his account of how events unfolded:

> One day, Dr. Edward B. Cragin, head obstetrician and gynecologist at the Sloane Hospital . . . telephoned me asking that I come at once to the hospital to see him about a matter of greatest importance. When I arrived there, he said that he had a typhoid epidemic of more than twenty cases on his hands. The other servants had joking nick-named (a) cook 'Typhoid Mary'. She was out at the moment, but would I recognize her handwriting if she really was that woman? He handed me a letter, from which I saw at once that the cook was indeed Mary Mallon, and I also identified her from his description. I advised that the Health Department be notified, and it was not long before Mary was again taken and sent to North Brother Island.

This account, which places Dr. Soper again at the center of things (and expands his ever-growing resume of talents to now include forensic handwriting expert), reeks of methane. Soper's insistence that he suggested that

Dr. Cragin 'notify the Health Department' is particularly ludicrous. The concept of typhoid carriers was old news now. The tracking of cases and analysis of samples was routine. Sloane Hospital – Soper seems not to notice – employed more than a few doctors, many of whom were victims of the outbreak. To make Soper's account even more unlikely, at the very time that the outbreak occurred a rigorous blind testing of typhoid vaccine was being conducted on doctors, nurses, and personnel at Sloane. Stool and urine samples were routinely being collected with an eye for positive results. That Soper would be contacted before the Health Department – or even considered in any official way – is absurd on its face.

Newspaper accounts of the day do not support Soper's version. Tests, it is said in the press, were in fact administered by a Dr. Norris L. Ogan of the Health Department. Mary Mallon, *still working* at the hospital after the outbreak was discovered, supplied stool samples, as did every other cook and servant and employee. When the results came back, revealing trace amounts of typhoid in her sample, she was soon no where to be found.

Dr. Soper was not alone in claiming to have tracked down Mary Mallon, Public Enemy Number One. Dr. Josephine Baker claimed later to have recognized Mary in the hospital kitchen, 'among the pots and pans'. A *New Yorker* magazine article written years later states that Dr. Baker 'notified the police and health authorities' and that 'that afternoon, when Mary left the hospital, she was followed. She had wrapped up a bowl of gelatin which she had lovingly prepared with her own lethal hands, and was taking it to the home of a friend who lived in Corona.'

Newspaper accounts, crediting Mary's discovery to the hospital stool sample, say she was tracked 'through friends' after going into hiding at the Corona address – a much more credible scenario. The story of Mary, caught in the act, about to deliver a 'lethal' bowl of gelatin to a friend, sounds like someone trying way too hard to build suspense into a rather humdrum account. It is more than likely that Mary's capture was the result of a friend giving her up. That's the way most fugitives are caught.

This didn't prevent a Sergeant Bevins on the New York Police Department from claiming that he had, in the course of his duties, recognized by 'her walk' a veiled Mary Mallon walking into a Corona home, and called in reinforcements.

However they got there, it came down to this: Sergeant Bevins, his lieutenant, Belton, another police sergeant, named Coneally, and 'various interested parties,' including Dr. Westmoreland (no mention of Soper or Baker), surrounded the Corona house. Sergeant Coneally rang the front doorbell. No answer. He rang again. No response. A ladder was found and Sergeant Coneally climbed to a window on the second floor and stuck his head into a dark room. A bulldog barked, provoking a fast retreat. The intrepid cop came down the ladder, found some meat with which to distract the intimidating pooch. Up the ladder again, followed by Bevins and others. They heard the sounds of doors being shut, one after another, and they followed.

In a bathroom, they found her. Typhoid Mary Mallon, crouching on the tile floor. She didn't struggle. She gave up without a fight. It was the end of the road.

She had known it was coming. She had had to know. Working at Sloane, in Manhattan, amongst doctors – some of whom were in the middle of extensive typhoid vaccine trials – was an insane risk, a desperate venture. The other cooks had even teased her, called her 'Typhoid Mary' – never dreaming she actually was. It was only a joke, yes, but one would picture an earlier, more energetic Mary Mallon taking that as a cue to leave. When she'd heard – as she must have – that the kitchen staff would be tested, she hadn't run. She had supplied a sample. Knowing the possible result, she hadn't bugged out for the sticks, avoided her usual haunts, or called a lawyer. She'd halfheartedly hidden in a bathroom when they came – and when confronted, had given up without a peep.

She was older now. And broken. Three years of imprisonment, living a convict's rules: eating when they told her to eat, sleeping when they told her to sleep, followed by five years in the culinary hinterlands, scrounging a living in bottom-rung jobs, one-lung rooming houses, taking orders from God knows what kind of despotic taskmasters. Those private homes where she might briefly have found employ, were most certainly not of the caliber she'd once enjoyed. To cook in the lower rungs of domestic service was not the same. The number of other servants were necessarily fewer. Cooking functions would be combined with the less glamorous tasks of laundry, cleaning, and scullery. The food would not have been as good, the masters less lovely, less generous. Who knows what she must have endured, what boorish and despotic bosses, flaky housemistresses, whining, inept servant girls, speaking to her with rudeness and contempt. She was tired. She was old. And she was guilty.

It's a measure of how little she cared about herself or anybody else that she would risk infecting pregnant women and newborn children with typhoid. It was . . . well . . . indefensible. Even taking a small chance that she could infect an infant or nursing mother with typhoid was contemptuous and contemptible. That she clearly couldn't even be bothered to wash her hands carefully after going to the bathroom – an easy measure, the least she could have done even if she was teeming with typhoid – speaks volumes about how far she had fallen and how little she cared.

Soper, in a smug but relatively sympathetic (for him) examination of subsequent events, says:

Mary was now about 48 years of age and a good deal heavier than she was when she slipped through a kitchen full of servants, jumped a back fence, and put up a fight

with strong, young policemen. She was as strong as ever,
but had lost something of that remarkable energy and
activity which had characterized her young days and
urged her forward undaunted. In those eight years since
she was first arrested, she had learned what it was to yield
to other wills than her own and to know pain. In the last
five years, although she had been free, there had been
times when she had found it hard to fight her battles
unaided.

On North Brother Island the City offered her a
comfortable place to live – a place where she could cook
and sleep and read to her heart's content. Her old age
was provided for. There was a good hospital with doctors
nearby. She knew by experience that the people on the
island would be kind to her.

However she might have felt about it, it was back to the
island for Mary Mallon.

It was over. She'd done a terrible thing – and she knew
it. No newspapers would be writing friendly pieces about
her plight now. The babies and pregnant women she'd
risked infecting at Sloane made that unlikely in the
extreme. O'Neill was dead – not that he'd ever helped
all that much. Breihof was long gone. And there was,
maybe, the relief of knowing it was all over. Like the
murder suspect who falls asleep in the interrogation room
(a famously known indicator of guilt), she went limp, gave
in, let all wash over her, turned her fate over to the

warders. No more hope – but no more worries. Her life of toil was over. No more scrounging, no more hustling, no more fear. The worst, finally, had happened. She was now, really and truly, away for life.

Chapter Eleven

Life Without

IN MARCH 1915, Mary Mallon was returned to North Brother Island. She would live there until she died – twenty-three years later. This time, she didn't fight it. She returned to her one-room bungalow and watched, begrudgingly but resignedly, as the world passed her by. Until the end, she refused to admit to others that she had in any way caused typhoid. She never discussed it – or allowed it to be discussed in her presence. Even with friends, she was close mouthed to the end – about her past, about her friends, about her personal life. Seemingly resigned to her fate, she kept herself busy sewing, crocheting, and by some accounts, baking cakes which she sold to other women on the island. Presumably, any bacteria she might have spread would be eliminated during the cooking process – but it seems an extraordinary leap of faith on the part of her customers.

She reacquainted herself with a nurse at Riverside, an Adelaide Offspring, and there were others who were kind to her and with whom she socialized. Offspring, judging from the amount Mary eventually left her in her will, was Mary's closest friend. They were seen walking and talking together many times – though what they discussed and the nature of their relationship remains unknown. Riverside Hospital, while it may have been remote – and the circumstances of her admission uncongenial – was, by standards of the time, an island of compassion. As a TB facility at a time when little could be done for those suffering from the disease, it employed doctors who were used to offering sympathy and kindness in place of as yet undiscovered medication. Dr. John Cahill, who ran the hospital during this final period of Mary Mallon's life, was remembered by his son, Dr. Kevin Cahill, as saying, 'What did you do before there were drugs? Before there were antibiotics? . . . You learned to sit on the bedside and hold the hand . . . every once in a while you gave the person a hug.'

Emma Goldberg Sherman, a bacteriologist, described for the BBC, getting off the boat at Riverside for the first time: 'This is heaven . . . it's delightful . . . otherworldly . . . unlike New York City.' She'd landed a job at another facility, but an anti-Semitic boss put the brakes on her employment there, telling her the position 'had been filled'. Riverside Hospital, on the other hand, was delighted to have her. Sherman talked for the cameras about what happened when she first came ashore at North Brother Island:

I walked into that building and climbed the stairs, a huge empty room with lots of tables standing around . . . and a huge woman in there who kind of terrified me with her

hair unkempt pulled back in a tight knot and a huge lab
coat which enfolded her despite her size at least double to
the floor – filthy as hell with all kinds of stuff on it.
And they told me this was Mary Mallon.

Sherman, who worked with her for some time and
seems to have been a sympathetic acquaintance – if not a
friend –was clearly repulsed by Mallon's personal hygiene.
She is not ambiguous in relating her first impression that
Mary was horrifyingly sloppy and unclean. Perhaps Mary's
relative size and rather imposing appearance gave her
pause. The small Sherman appears in a rare photograph
with Mary, and Mary, much older and larger now than in
earlier depictions, does tower over the bacteriologist. In
the photo Mary's hair is shown pulled back so tightly it
looks like a man's, her skin wattled under a thick neck,
fists balled under the too-long sleeves of a voluminous lab
coat. She is squinting through clear glasses, her mouth
drooping slightly on one side – either from, as Judith
Leavitt postulates, an early minor stroke, or from her bad
teeth (which she would not allow hospital dentists to look
at). In the picture she appears big, scary, sexless and . . .
proud. Her back is stiff, her arms are at her sides, and while
that may not be a real smile on her face, it is not a look of
displeasure. Mary is posing for the camera in her work
clothes – with her colleague – and she looks glad to be
working. Says Sherman uncharitably:

She centrifuged urine . . . Though what she saw when she looked through the microscope I don't know . . . She knew nothing. Absolutely nothing. I think she contaminated everything she touched . . . When it came to washing the bottles . . . well . . . what the hell.

Her first show of friendship to me she came up from one of her visits . . . and brought me this exquisite apple . . . she was rubbing her hands . . . and well . . . her hands were tremendous. She was a big woman and she managed to cover every piece of that poor apple. She presented it to me – What do I do with it? I didn't want to eat it. I didn't even want to touch it!

Sherman tells how she placed the gift deliberately close to a centrifuge, making sure to contaminate it with spilled fluid so she could discreetly dispose of the gift without offending her assistant. She later threw the apple out.

Others at the hospital still referred to Mary as 'Typhoid Mary', but only behind her back. No one called her that to her face, and all were careful to not raise the subject in front of her. Some maintain that she would fly into a rage if the matter of typhoid was discussed in her presence – but maybe they were just frightened of the imposing-looking woman and her reputation. She was still bitter about the forces which had put her on the island – still claiming she'd been the undeserved target of evil doctors, without justification. From time to time, she wrote threatening letters to Dr. Baker and Dr. Biggs. In her bungalow, she kept the shades and curtains drawn, to keep out prying eyes.

'There never seemed to be any youth in her,' says Emma Sherman. She still never discussed her past, never reminisced about old loves, fondly recalled picnics or her childhood.

> She must have had fun. She must have had friends. She must have gone around places with people. There was never any mention that she did. She was very, very closemouthed.

In 1918, the hospital began allowing Mary to make day trips off the island unsupervised.

'She never told me where she went when she went off the island. Always back the same day', says Sherman.

One place she went was to the home of Dr. Alexandra Plavska. Another likely destination was the home of Mary Lempe, a friend in Woodside who had apparently put her up during her time on the run. She always dressed 'very fashionably', according to Sherman, though, other witnesses claim, always in black. Black dress, black shawl, black stockings and black shoes. 'She looked very substantial.' Though Sherman was curious, she never questioned her. 'What am I going to ask her? "Who's your boyfriend?" I wasn't going to ask her, "Were you ever married?"'

Dr. Plavska, like Adelaide Offspring, was as close a

friend as Mary had during this last period of her life. Plavska was (it is said) a countess, who had graduated from the school of medicine at Moscow University in 1917. When she arrived at Riverside in 1925, she gave Mary a job as her lab assistant. As Mary had apparently been doing less than stellar work with Sherman, one can only assume that this was make-work – a kindness on the part of Dr. Plavska – as must have been her previous work. Mary was a frequent visitor to Plavska's home in the years during her work with the doctor and for years after.

Julie Efros, Plavska's granddaughter, says:

She would bring little things. She was very beholden to my grandmother. My grandmother was a baroness. They became good friends . . . she felt flattered that she was part of the family. And we really loved her.

She looked like a man . . . We'd scrub the dishes and boil the dishes when she had dinner with us. She was warm and dear and was always trying to help in some way.

In the BBC documentary, Efros speaks warmly of Mary as a beloved friend. At one point, she remembers a crocheted shawl which Mary gave her and models it for the camera. What did they talk about at these gatherings, the countess-turned-doctor, the little girl and the notorious Mary Mallon?

Maybe life wasn't so bad, considering.

Mary Mallon, during the worst years of the Great Depression, had her own home, a paying job, and the freedom, at least, to visit friends, shop, sightsee as she wished. She had little money, but few did in those days. Many of her peers in the domestic cooking trade were probably faring much, much worse out in the world as jobs dried up and the rich became less rich and the poor starved. It was hardly a resort she was living in – but by Depression era standards, it was a warm, dry, secure home, with three squares a day, free medical care should she have wanted it, a paying job and leisure time. As retirement facilities went, not too shabby. Not that this was much comfort.

In December 1932, Emma Sherman noticed that Mary was late to work in the lab. She had never been late before and Sherman became worried for her. She walked over to Mary's bungalow.

The stench that came out of that doorway . . . It was dark, because she never raised the curtains . . . grimy, filthy-looking on the outside . . . I called and there was no answer. I knocked. So I pushed the door open. I could barely get it open because there was so much junk . . . I almost slid into the place it was so filthy. The odor was overwhelming. There she was . . . lying [on the floor] moaning . . . I couldn't get near her . . . I just couldn't – it was a physical impossibility with all the stuff that was around.

She had had a paralyzing stroke. When Sherman saw her later in her hospital bed, she saw that Mary's face appeared to be smiling. The stroke had distorted her appearance, making her look like she was frozen in a grimace. Mary looked at Sherman and took her to be Betty Compton, the one-time girlfriend of Mayor Jimmy Walker. She 'didn't know who I was', says Sherman. But, 'I kept seeing her regularly for a long time.' After a while, dismayed that Mary still could not even recognize her, Sherman, who had by now left the island, stopped visiting entirely. 'There was no point.' Mary remained bedridden for the next six years, a prisoner now not only of North Brother Island, but of her own flesh. In 1933, five years before she died, Mary Mallon dictated her will to a lawyer.

Dr. Plavska and granddaughter Julie continued visiting Mary in her hospital bed until the end. Mary remembered the kindness of Dr. Plavska and her family with a final bequest of 200 dollars when she died on November 11, 1938. She left another 200 to the Lempe family and 250 to St. Luke's Church in the Bronx where her funeral was held. She left a rather astonishing sum of over 4000 dollars, the bulk of her estate, to Adelaide Offspring. She had clearly saved much of the money she'd made on the island. She paid for her own gravestone. Nine people attended her funeral; the Lempe family, the Plavskas, and Nurse Offspring are the only ones named (numbering seven). As far as we know, no one from the Health Department or from any city agency showed up.

Mary was buried in St. Raymond's Cemetery in the Bronx. The gravestone inscription reads:

Mary Mallon
Died Nov 11 1938
JESUS MERCY

Epilogue

Goodbyes

IT SEEMED ONLY RIGHT to go see her, the woman I'd been reading about, writing about, thinking about for the last year. I thought a token of appreciation would be nice – a gesture, however late and futile.

I tried to get out to North Brother Island first, wanting to see for myself what it must have looked like from out there. Easier said than done. Getting a boat to take me out, regardless of bribes and inducements offered, was not doable in the time I had. The Coast Guard obligingly offered to take me, but canceled at the very last minute, claiming engine trouble. It was a very cold day in December with high winds, choppy swells in the river – and I couldn't blame them even if they had simply decided it was better to stay ashore than lug some writer upriver to a deserted island and wait around in very tricky current where the Sound meets the river while he communes with the dead. I settled for a drive in the Bronx, down Fordham road, to the parking lot of a warehouse, where I stood by the shore and peered out over the water to the island only a few hundred yards away.

There's a tantalizing and odd fragment on the Internet, some Web site where it is claimed that a portal to another world exists on the island in one of the moldering old structures that once comprised Riverside Hospital. An opening between walls, where some persistent true believer in Bigfoot, Living Elvis and Parallel Universes has painted a mural, decorating some imagined psychic transporter made of crumbling plaster. Empty rooms.

The cottage where Mary lived the last years of her life before her stroke is gone. But much of the hospital apparently remains, however ruined. I don't know what I could have learned there, but I'm sorry I missed it. It's an ominous sight, the island, especially in the harsh, gray light of winter – something a screenwriter or a novelist might describe as 'brooding'. The tops of chimneys or smokestacks poke through overgrown trees and underbrush; dark shapes are seen through branches. A not-very-confidence-inspiring concrete mooring seems to sag into the water. In the distance, Riker's Island looks positively cheery by comparison. It's the end of the world. While the city and its skyline have certainly changed since Mary's time there, the island can hardly have become much lovelier. It's a Godforsaken piece of rock in the middle of nowhere. From where I was standing, the greenish water lapping at mossy stones, I could see discarded crack vials, used condoms, a doll's head. The other shores looked no more inviting. On this day there were no pleasure boats. A single freighter scudded by on the way to the Sound, and that was it. I was glad to leave.

Thirty-third and Third, where Mary shacked up with

Breihof, where Soper confronted her on the stairs, looks completely different from the old photographs of the site taken back in her day. No ghosts linger. The Third Avenue el, which must have rumbled noisily past her window as she snored in bed, her dog and her man close at hand, is long, long gone. All of New York's got history. You can barely walk a block without passing the scene of a long-ago tragedy, a mob execution, the last resting place of a famous writer, a place you once scored or groped an old girlfriend, a one-time speakeasy, a KGB money drop, a place with freakish significance. Most now are just patches of concrete, somehow drained of soul over time.

I visited my mom in a hospital room on the exact site of Mary's last place of employ. (It was nothing serious – a one-day visit.) It's a different hospital now, a different world. A glimmer of recognition and wonder still tingles the senses when one walks through the Waldorf Astoria lobby – a place where Mary would hardly have been welcome, but where her masters undoubtedly visited and played. Madison Square is unrecognizable, the Flatiron building emanates something – but that's probably because my publisher operates out of it – and I have yet to finish this manuscript. The old Luchows on Fourteenth Street, where I once visited during its brief revival as a nightclub, left a lasting impression – as did Keen's steakhouse – both places where one can easily imagine Diamond Jim and Lillian Russell stuffing their faces. Did Mary ever get a good meal in a fancy restaurant? Did Breihof ever clean up a bit, throw on a suit, and take her out for a dance and some fine food, a couple of cocktails? I still don't know.

The territory of feared street gangs, opium rings, white slavers, the tenement districts where Irish immigrants once lived, are expensive neighborhoods now. The Lower East Side looks like a theme park – a Disney recreation of urban living for the young, white and wealthy. Hell's Kitchen is worse, the shabby burlesque houses and night-clubs and porno houses of even a few years back replaced by theme restaurants, merchandising outlets for the WWF and Warner Brothers.

The Holland Tunnel inspires awe, still. It's hard not to imagine the amazement when it first opened, what an engineering miracle it must have seemed – even in a time filled with engineering miracles.

Oyster Bay? Dark Harbor? Tuxedo Park? Blur your eyes and pretend – and maybe, depending on where you're standing, you can get a sense of what they looked like then.

St. Raymond's Cemetery, in the Bronx, Mary's final resting place, still has a powerful effect. I went up there in the freezing cold. Dead leaves blew dramatically over the acres of headstones. It took some doing, finding her headstone. They did a lot of dying in 1938, and most of the company around her passed on that same year. The names on the stones are immigrant names, Irish, Italian, a few Slavs and Germans. Plenty of history where Mary lays. Fat Tony Salerno is buried there. It's where the ransom money for the Lindbergh baby was dropped. Mary's gravestone, which she paid for herself, is simple and relatively undecorated, looking like thousands of others nearby. The pattern cut into the stone is unremarkable, and the inscription, JESUS MERCY, as tempting as it might be to infer as evidence of a guilty conscience, is the same as hundreds of others, along with REST IN PEACE, and a score of other Hallmark-style sentiments. In Mary's case, looking at it, the two words seem particularly personal, as if she herself was saying them. No DEARLY BELOVED or WE WILL ALWAYS REMEMBER YOU, signifying that loved ones remained. Hers, however ubiquitous in the poetry of the dead, reads as plaintive. A last cry for good fortune, better luck, salvation.

The ground is soft in spots at St. Raymond's. Approaching her headstone, my foot pushed through the topsoil and plunged to the knee into soft, brittle earth. I didn't want to get that close to her. I apologized to her neighbor for nearly stepping on his face and stood for a long time in front of her grave. I'd brought her a present.

In 1973, I bought my first chef's knife, a high-carbon Sabatier with a polished wooden handle. I was so proud of it – and I've held onto it all these years, remembering how it felt in my hand when I first unwrapped it, the way the handle rested against my palm, the feel of the blade, the sharpness of the edge. It's old now, and stained, and the handle is cracked slightly in spots. I long ago gave up using it or trying to maintain it. But it is a beloved object.

Something a fellow cook would appreciate, I hoped – a once fine hunk of quality French steel – a magical fetish, a beloved piece of my personal history. And a sign of respect, I hoped, an indicator that somebody, somewhere, even long after her troubles and her dying, took her seriously, understood, if only a little bit, the difficulty of her life as a cook. It's the kind of gift I would like to receive, one that I would understand.

I looked around the graveyard, making sure that no one else was watching, leaned over and with my hands, pulled back the grass at the base of her stone. I slipped my knife down there, covered it up the way it had looked before and left it for her. It was the least I could do.

A gift. Cook to cook.

Bibliography/Suggested Reading

Batterberry, Michael and Ariane. *On the Town in New York*. Routledge, 1999.

Bayor, Ronald, and Timothy J. Meagher, eds. *The New York Irish*. Johns Hopkins Press, 1996.

Botkin, B.A. *New York City Folklore*. Random House.

Byron, Joseph. *New York Life at the Turn of the Century in Photographs*. Dover Publications, 1985.

Cahill, Kevin, M.D., ed. *The American Irish Revival: A Decade of the Recorder – 1974–1983*. Associated Faculty Press.

Chambers, Julius. *The Book of New York: 40 Years of Recollections of the American Metropolis*. 1912.

Mrs. Child. *The American Frugal Housewife*. Carter Hendee and Co., 1833.

Crockett, Albert Stevens. *Peacocks on Parade: A Narrative of a Unique Period in American Social History and Its Most Colorful Figures*. 1931.

Deshon, Rev. George. *Guide for Catholic Young Women: Especially Those Who Earn Their Own Living*. Catholic Book Exchange.

Ellis, Edward Robb. *The Epic of New York City*. Kodansha, 1997.

Federspiel, J.F. *The Ballad of Typhoid Mary*.

Gordon, Richard. *Famous and Difficult Patients: Amusing Medical Anecdotes from Typhoid Mary to FDR*. St. Martin's Press.

Groneman, Carol, and Mary Beth Norton, eds. *To Toil the Livelong Day: America's Women at Work 1780–1980*. Cornell University Press.

Holt, Hamilton, ed. *The Life Stories of Undistinguished Americans As Told by Themselves*. Routledge.

James, Henry. *New York Revisited*. Franklin Square Press, 1994.

Kouwenhoven, John A. *The Columbia Historical Portrait of New York*. Icone Editions, Harper and Row, 1953.

Leavitt, Judith Walzer. *Typhoid Mary: Captive To The Public's Health*. Beacon Press, 1996.

Levenstein, Harvey. *Revolution at the Table*. Oxford University Press, 1988.

Markel, Howard. *When Germs Travel*. The American Scholar, Spring 1999.

Seitz, Sharon, and Stuart Miller. *The Other Islands of New York City*. Countryman Press.

Mitchell, Joseph. *Up in the Old Hotel*. Vintage Books, 1993.

Plante, Ellen M. *The American Kitchen: 1700 to Present*. Facts On File, 1995.

Ranhofer, Charles. *The Epicurean: A Complete Treatise of Analytical and Practical Studies on the Culinary Art*. New York, 1903.

Rosenberg, Charles E. *The Cholera Years: The United States in 1832, 1849 and 1866*.

Sante, Luc. *Low Life*. Vintage, 1990.

Soper, George A., Ph.D. *The Curious Career of Typhoid Mary*. Delivered before the Section of Historical and Cultural Medicine, New York Academy of Medicine, and published in the Bulletin of the Academy, Oct. 1939.

Stansell, Christine. *City of Women: Sex and Class in New York*. University of Illinois Press, 1987.

Wilkes, Roger, ed. *The Mammoth Book of Unsolved Crimes*. Carrol and Graf.

Acknowledgements

Thanks to: Hope Killcoyne for her dogged and spectacular research on a difficult subject. Joel Rose, Gladys Bourdain (thanks, Mom), Michael Batterberry, the incredible Rose Marie Morse at Morse Partners. Brian Anderson. Assistant Comissioner of Geneology and Public Relations at the New York City Department of Records and Information Services, Ken Cobb, Bill Cobert of the Irish Historical Society, Dr. Kevin Cahill, Clem Berne, Melinda Gellman, Dimitri Kasterine. Maureen Hope. Peter Herb and Andrea Moss (legal documents). Jonothan Kuhn, Director of Arts and Antiquities for the New York City Parks Department, Ellen Morales at the Museum of the City of New York, Rebecca Tatem and Scott Norman at the BBC, Ed O'Donnel, The New York Historical Society – particularly Juliet Berman, Kathleen Hulser and the photo and library departments, the staff at the New York Public Library Reference and Microfilm departments. Lisa Westheimer. Paul Paradise of the Municipal Reference and Research Center, Bonnie Slotnick, Meryle Evans, Matt and Tracy at Kitchen Arts and Letters, my brother, Chris Bourdain, for getting me out to St. Raymond's Cemetary and helping all the way. Kim Witherspoon.

Camelia Cassin. Philippe Lajaunie and Jose de Meireilles at Les Halles. Edilberto Perez, sous-chef extraordinaire, Pascal Graf, chef de cuisine (for covering my ass in the kitchen) and to all the chefs and line cooks I've met in the last ridiculous and wonderful year. You know you you are.

A Note on the Author

Anthony Bourdain is the author of *Kitchen Confidential: Adventures in the Culinary Underbelly*, and the novels *Bone in the Throat* and *Gone Bamboo*. He is the executive chef at Brasserie Les Halles in New York City.

A Note on the Type

The text of this book is set in Linotype Goudy
Old Style. It was designed by Frederic Goudy
(1865–1947), an American designer whose types
were very popular during his lifetime, and particularly
fashionable in the 1940s. He was also a craftsman who
cut the metal patterns for his type designs, engraved
matrices and cast type.

The design for Goudy Old Style is based on Goudy
Roman, with which it shares a 'hand-wrought'
appearance and asymmetrical serifs, but unlike
Goudy Roman its capitals are modelled on
Renaissance lettering.